Hands-On
Activities for Children
with Autism
& Sensory
Disorders

Recipes   Crafts   Exercises   Sensory Enrichment
Multisensory Immersion   For Home, School, Clinic

Teresa Garland, MOT, OTR/L
Bestselling author of *Self-Regulation Interventions and Strategies*

"Teresa Garland has captured the essence of using the occupation of play to enrich the lives of the children we all adore. Having several years of experience working with children diagnosed with Autism, and sensory disorders, I have a solid appreciation for effective practice. Teresa manages to expound upon evidence-based strategies packaged for parents, teachers, and therapists alike. Her book encompasses techniques draped in the strongest aspects of sensory, gross motor, and emotional approaches. It is a beautiful arrangement that allows the reader to apply aspects of occupational therapy, and related fields, to simplistic and enjoyable activities. Teresa continues to contribute to our field by translating and demystifying therapeutic strategies to everyday life!"

-Dr. Varleisha D. Gibbs OTR/L
Author, Expert Speaker

"Teresa Garland has done it again! Another excellent activity book that provides detailed treatment protocols with amazing visuals and hands-on activities for therapists to use with children with sensory impairments."

-Cara Marker Daily, PhD
Pediatric Psychologist

"Anyone involved in the life of a child who has autism or a sensory modulation disorder will treasure this resource. Ms. Garland has done the heavy lifting to produce a detailed, accessible guide with fresh and practical sensory activities. Especially helpful are her recommendations for grading activities from very simple to more complex. These activities will not only revitalize interventions for therapists but also equip motivated do-it-yourself parents to engage in sensory learning with their children."

-Sheryl Ryan, PhD, OTR/L

"I learned so much!"

-Candace E. Edwards, MS, OTR

Published by
PESI Publishing & Media
PESI, Inc
3839 White Ave
Eau Claire, WI 54703

Cover: Amy Rubenzer
Layout: Bookmasters & Amy Rubenzer

ISBN: 9781559570695

Printed in the United States of America.

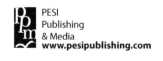

PESI
Publishing
& Media
www.pesipublishing.com

Acknowledgements

I'm grateful to Linda Jackson and her publishing staff at PESI—Karsyn Morse, Hillary Jenness, and Amy Rubenzer.

Many people graciously helped to coordinate the photo shoots: Jana Ripaska, MS, OTR, and Dean Jennifer Hoppesch at Plymouth Scholars in Plymouth, Michigan; Stephanie Naberhaus, Joanie Davidson Forfinski, and Janice Pagano at Building Bridges Therapy Center; and the staff at PROCAM in Livonia, Michigan. Sarah Grosjean assisted with the studio photo shoot.

Many children patiently and generously posed for photos: Devin Allen, Ethan Ayers, Ava Azzouz, Aidan Brown, Bradley Caloia, Christopher Caloia, Alijah Door, Adam Funk, Liam Gibbons, Daniel Grosjean, Faith Grosjean, Lawrence Grosjean, Noah Hansen, Sean Harvey, Dylan Heasley, Jacob Heintzleman, Luke Humphreys, Amelia Kumor, Max Kumor, Victoria Maes, Justin Marcarian, Grace Murdock, Halaya Reynolds, Stephan Russo, Isaac Schmitt, Lily Stewart, Max Stewart, and Kaylin Valli.

Building Bridges Therapy Center in Plymouth granted me generous access to facilities, staff and clients for the photo shoots. Therapists there generously gave of their time and creativity: Candace Edwards, MS, OTR; Jana Repaska, MS, OTR; Ann Moro-Hill, MS, OTR; and Jean Walsh, SLP-CCC. Jean also advised me on speech-and-language related activities for the mix-ins chapter and generously shared materials including a list of read-aloud children's books.

Thanks to readers Sheryl Ryan, PhD, OTR/L, Joshua Brown, DOT, OTR/L, Candace Edwards, MS, OTR/L and Jana Ripaska, MS, OTR/L. A special thanks to Stephanie Ramser, OTR, for her help with the material in Chapter 2, Jana Repaska who inspired the sensory-immersion chapters, and Sarah Repasky for helping me locate recipes, instructions and materials, and for her encouragement along the way.

Two researchers were incredibly generous in allowing me to use their work: Dr. Michael Leon gave permission to run with the Environmental Enrichment protocol and Jasmine Ma gave permission to use her FUNtervals routines.

Last but not least, thanks to my husband, Peter Michaelson, for his loving support throughout the writing process.

Table of Contents

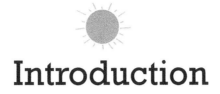

Introduction

This book is filled with an abundance of fun, hands-on activities for children. The activities will help reduce symptoms of sensory modulation disorder (SMD), and at the same time induce pleasure. The activities, crafts, poems, recipes and exercises within these pages are intended to bring a big smile to the face of the sensory child and allow her to relax and think—and feel—that "Life is good!"

This book aims to increase the sensory regulation skills of children with SMD and children with autism spectrum disorder (ASD). The book's four key approaches are to:

1. Educate the sensory systems of children with ASD via a six-month protocol created by Woo & Leon (2015) called Environmental Enrichment. This protocol, detailed and annotated in this book, has been found to be effective in children with ASD. The protocol trains the child's brain to recognize and utilize multi-sensory environmental input including touch, smell, sound, vision and balance. In one study (Woo, 2015), 21 percent of children who completed the protocol shed ASD symptoms to the degree that they lost their ASD label (although they retained enough symptoms to still be on the spectrum.) Other children who did not lose their label still made significant gains in reducing the severity of autism.

2. Desensitize the child with SMD and ASD to noxious environmental input. Several specific desensitization techniques are covered in the book, with examples in the areas of sound, touch, taste and smell sensitivities. There is also a general discussion of desensitization that will help the reader to adapt these techniques to other areas.

3. Immerse the child in pleasant sensory input. The book provides fun, sensory-based activities that give him the sensory input he needs. At the same time, the child is taught skills that are useful for establishing sensory-based hobbies through engagement with the sensory aspects of a variety of materials such as clay, yarns, metal and music. Activities include several long projects that can be completed over several weeks, as well as multi-sensory projects.

4. Regulate the child through intensive exercise. The book contains fun, yet strenuous movement activities designed by Jasmine Ma and appropriately named FUNtervals. Instructions for creating your own FUNtervals are also given.

Why is an enrichment program important? Studies indicate that between five to sixteen percent of all children have significant problems processing sensory input, to the degree that they qualify for a diagnosis of SMD. That percentage compares to that of children diagnosed with attention deficit hyperactivity disorder (ADHD), yet SMD doesn't receive the same attention because children with SMD tend to be better behaved and have better functional skills in the classroom.

SMD symptoms include a combination of oversensitivity to sensory input, undersensitivity to sensory input, and may also produce cravings for certain sensations. The symptoms vary with the child. Children with SMD struggle to keep body, mind (attention) and emotions self-regulated. For a sensitive child, the symptoms can be acute and very disturbing. Environmental sounds, physical touch, and internal sensation such as pain and temperature register acutely in the brain and can sometimes provoke a fight-flight response. The opposite is true for the undersensitive child who misses out on some of the pleasures in life and is at higher risk for injury. Pain expert and fibromyalgia researcher, Dr. Dan Clauw, compares sensory sensitivity in the brain to a sound system in which the amps are turned up too loud. Similarly, we can think of undersensitivity as amps that are turned down too low. It goes without saying, a child with these symptoms is often an unhappy child—and perhaps quite cranky, too. Fortunately, as that child gets older, she slowly learns to live with the amps turned up or down. And around the age of eight, her abstract reasoning skills emerge and she is able to develop coping strategies. She knows when and where not to pick battles about the things that irritate. She also tends to suffer in silence when she has no control over her environment.

While we don't have a cure for the symptoms that plague children with SMD, there's much we can do to reduce symptoms and help children live with them. In fact, life with SMD is not all bad. The person who is oversensitive to noise, for example, is also very sensitive to music and might experience a wonderful sense of joy from listening to it. The person who craves sensation might find a career as a cook, artist or mechanic. And the person with undersensitivity might become laid-back and more immune to life's stressors.

The premise of this book is that the sensory child can learn to put suffering aside and be happy and well-regulated. To that end, this book provides techniques to help desensitize the child to touch, taste and sound, and to give the child who craves sensory input activities that immerse him in pleasant sensory sensation, helping him to be at ease.

This book also provides techniques to improve sensory functionality of children with ASD. Lane (2014) found that 62 percent of children with ASD have moderate-to-severe sensory processing problems. Ten percent of these children have sensitivity to body sensation, including issues with posture and core strength; 40 percent have extreme taste and smell sensitivities; and 12 percent have overall sensory dysfunction. As well, most children with ASD have difficulty processing speech, especially when competing background noises are present. They also crave touching things. Sensory symptoms in a child with ASD can be so severe as to compromise basic sensory function. For example, a child may have extraordinarily sensitive touch, or poor registration of temperature or pain.

Sensory symptoms can interact with and exacerbate symptoms of autism such as poor joint-attention and poor attention to environmental cues, resulting in the child fixating on objects such as fans and clocks and not performing work in the classroom. For children with autism, poor attention to the environment might also cause a fight-flight reaction when something unexpected happens. Their poor verbal skills make it difficult for them to let others know their displeasure with bright lights, loud noises, or someone touching them. Poor verbal skills also limit their ability to assume functional control in those situations. This, in turn, may lead to behavioral overreactions. Adults may then inadvertently address the behavior, leading to unsatisfactory outcomes, rather than the underlying sensory factors.

To improve such a child's ability to process environmental input, we must first build a foundation for him by training his brain to recognize basic sensory input such as: this is warm; this is cool; this is hot; this is cold. A program for building that foundation exists, and it has been found to be quite effective for children with autism, helping them to shed symptoms of autism and improve sensory processing and verbal reception skills. The program, Environmental Enrichment, is detailed in this book. The program is an excellent first step in educating the senses. Again, it does not resolve all symptoms of SMD, but improves them. Children doing the program will also benefit from the techniques mentioned earlier, namely desensitization and immersion in sensory activities (Woo, 2013, 2015).

Sections and Chapters

The book comprises three sections that cover these topics: 1) information for the therapist, teacher and parent regarding sensory modulation and tips for working with children with SMD, 2) a complete implementation guide for the Environmental Enrichment protocol (for children with ASD), and 3) fun techniques for helping children work through symptoms of SMD. Below is an outline of those sections and the chapters within them.

The first section covers the basics of doing sensory-based interventions with children, including **children with autism**.

Chapter 1 provides foundational information about the senses, including how to screen for SMD, the types of problems that can occur, and general techniques for working with children with SMD.

Chapter 2 discusses the ten core elements for providing good interactive training to a child. The elements were identified by leading sensory experts as being especially effective for children with SMD or the overarching disorder, Sensory Processing Disorder. They are also helpful in guiding interventions for all children.

The second section is devoted to providing the Environmental Enrichment protocol to children of all ages with autism.

Chapter 3 provides background about the Environmental Enrichment program. Two variations are offered, a short version with 15 enrichment exercises, and a long version with 34 enrichment exercises. The two versions are individually described, and compared and contrasted. Instructions for performing the protocols are included in this chapter.

Chapter 4 details each of the 34 enrichment activities along with the materials list. In addition to Woo and Leon's protocol outline, there are activity instructions, photo illustrations and graded (both easier and harder) alternate activities designed by the author.

Chapter 5 contains additional foundation activities in the areas of speech, movement and emotions that can be done alongside the Environmental Enrichment program.

The third section covers the topic of sensory enrichment for children with and without autism.

Chapters 6 – 9 contain activities for touch desensitization and touch immersion; taste desensitization and scent immersion; sound desensitization and sound immersion; and visual immersion, respectively. The underlying goal is to regulate the child and to introduce him to the pleasures that can be had from his sensory systems. Each topic area begins with simple activities that teach basic sensory skills and craft skills. Activities become more complex and can involve long projects, such as making a 20-inch monkey from yarn and a multi-sensory sensory indoor planter.

Chapter 10 contains several intense movement activities, and it spells out how to create others. Included are several FUNtervals, the story-based high-intensity interval training routines that were developed by kinesiologist Jasmine Ma (2013, 2015).

Chapter 11 contains instructions for longer, more complex sensory immersion activities described in chapters 6-9.

How to Use This Book

You can make use of this book to:

- Discover new sensory activities to use with a child, a group of children or a whole classroom
- Implement an Environmental Enrichment program for a child with autism
- Implement a touch, sound or taste desensitization program
- Implement sensory immersion programs for a child with sensory sensitivity
- Find an intense movement activity for a child or a whole classroom
- Learn how to create your own intense movement activities

Using Programs Versus Single Activities

You may elect to do one of the formal or informal programs. Keep in mind that the book is packed with activities that can be used for sensory intervention independent of an overall program. The interventions in each topic area are graded by difficulty, making them easier to select. They range from very simple (in the Environmental Enrichment activities) through complex (the multi-sensory projects), and they cover a wide range of sensory needs for children. Below is a quick guide to exercises and activities. The tables are arranged by sense and by type of intervention (education, desensitization and immersion). Each table lists activities in the order of their difficulty and tells which chapter the activity is in. For example, in the touch education and desensitization table, 22 activities from four different chapters are listed. The activity numbers guide you to the location in the chapter.

Cold / Hot		
Chapter	Activity	Activity number
4	Hands, feet in bowls	1, 14
4	Coolness /warmth on skin	8, 9, 18
4	Play with cold items	12, 22
4	Carry cooled item	23
7	Drawing with food	3
6	Cook's helper	7

Emotional education		
Chapter	Activity	Activity number
5	Faces in the mirror	6
5	Name an emotion	7

Touch education and desensitization

Chapter	Activity	Activity number
4	Textured objects	2, 19, 20, 22
4	Draw lines on skin + texture	3, 5, 21
4	Matching objects blindfolded	8
4	Touch and manipulation	15, 25
4	Massage	24
9	Fabric swatches	2
7	Drawing with food	3
6	Desensitization to gooey things	1-6
6	Desensitization of food	7, 8
7	Scented dough	6

Touch immersion

Chapter	Activity	Activity number
6	Pipe cleaner activities	9
6	Simple yarn activities	10, 11, 12
6	Yarn projects	13, 14
6	Pebbles and glass bead projects	15, 16
6	Metal and coins	17-20
6	Simple wood activities	21, 22
6	Wood projects	23
6	Gooey immersion	24
9	Scented-fruit mobile	11
9	Collage with dried flowers	13

Visual education

Chapter	Activity	Activity number
4	Blindfold match, blindfold walk	4, 6, 11, 16
4	Matching	10, 12, 20, 31
4	Attention and tracking	13, 27, 33
4	Naming objects	17
4	Visual-auditory	34
8	Read books	3
9	Mosaic project	8

Visual immersion

Chapter	Activity	Activity number
6	Bunny, frog pictures	3, 5
9	Colors and coloring	1, 2
6	Sorting coins	18
6	Simple collage	4
7	Drawing with food	3
9	Stained glass	3
9	Paper strips and weaving	4, 5
9	Mosaics	6, 7, 8
6	Pebble mosaic	14
7	Pebble planter and plants	6
9	Fabric collage	9
6	Drawing with tools	17
9	Mobiles	10, 11
9	Collage projects	12, 13

Sound desensitization and education

Chapter	Activity	Activity number
4	Temperature	8
4	Distract from visual	13
4	Visual-auditory	34
4	Listen to music each day	In chapter 3
8	More music	2
8	Emotional reaction	1
5	Whistles blowing	1, 2
5	Make sounds	3, 4
5	Gestures	5
8	More gestures	4
8	Sound for desensitization	5

Sound immersion

Chapter	Activity	Activity number
8	Read special books	3
8	Make and use sound effects	5, 6
8	Rhymes	7, 8
5	Rhythm	9
8	Music	8

Scent immersion

Chapter	Activity	Activity number
9	Scented-fruit mobile	11
6	Play with scented dough	6
7	Make scented objects	Scent 1, Scent 2
7	Using scented herbs	Scent 3, Scent 4, Scent 5
7	Make an indoor garden	Scent 6

Scent education and food desensitization

Chapter	Activity	Activity number
4	Bath scent and oil	7
4	Smell odorant	In chapter 3
6	Play with scented dough	6
7	Eating activities	Food 1, Food 2, Food 3
6	Cook's helper	7
6	Birds' nests	8

Motor immersion

Chapter	Activity	Activity number
10	Popcorn FUNterval	1
10	Zoo FUNterval	2
10	Rock, paper, scissors FUNterval	3
10	Pirate hunt FUNterval	4
10	Make your own FUNterval	5

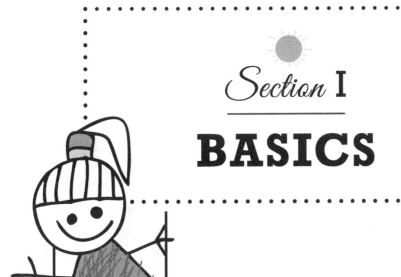

Section I

BASICS

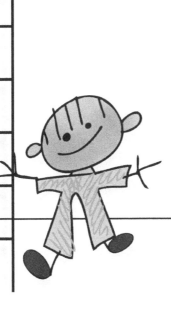

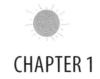

CHAPTER 1

Sensory Modulation Basics

Every second the brain processes an enormous amount of data that have been gathered by the skin, eyes, nose, tongue and ears and sent to the brain along nerve pathways. We also process a wide variety of internal body states that include muscle movement, balance, temperature, pain, gut sensations, and breath. Inside the brain, each sense organ's input is organized and encoded. Higher level circuitry identifies the sensation and decides whether to attend to it, store it, and share it with other senses and cognitive processes. This is "sensory processing," and when it is dysfunctional, we say that the person has a Sensory Processing Disorder (SPD).

Poor sensory processing is at the heart of many different functional problems that affect our ability to sense, identify and make use of external and internal sensations. It also affects our ability to coordinate our body movement (praxis). Attention and memory circuitry within each sense's cortical region can also fail, causing problems such as poor attention to visual tasks and poor auditory memory.

Sensory modulation, a subset of sensory processing, is concerned with each sense's degree of sensitivity (e.g., sensitivity to light touch) and with the brain's ability to regulate physical, mental and emotional reactions to sensory input. When a person is unable to regulate normal environmental sounds, light, smells and so on, we refer to the problem as poor sensory modulation. When people are highly dysfunctional in this regard, we say they have a Sensory Modulation Disorder (SMD). SMD includes three types of symptoms: over-responsivity, under-responsivity, and craving of sensory input. (I use the simpler terms, oversensitive, and undersensitive, to stand in place of over-responsive and under-responsive.) These symptoms can affect one or more of a person's senses. The three types of symptoms are independent problems, and so they can simultaneously occur in a single sense.

We are still in the early stages of understanding SMD's causes and how to assess and treat it. Let's take a brief look at what we know.

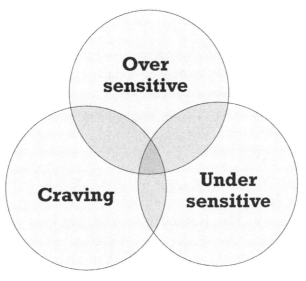

Oversensitivity comes from having a low threshold for sensation such as light, soft touch, noises, pain, aromas. Children with this problem become easily overwhelmed with sensation. Think of it as the "volume knob" on sensory input that is turned up too high, or as a lack of habituation to sensation. Acute oversensitivity can make social situations difficult to endure, as the examples below illustrate.

A child who is **undersensitive** doesn't register what others do. Although the problem is not generally emotionally disturbing, it can be dangerous. The child might have difficulty registering sensation such as smells, pain, temperature or balance, leading the child to be at risk for burns, injuries and falls. Without normal stimulation, the child can easily become bored, resulting in low alertness, inattention and sometimes sedentary behaviors. We can think of this problem as the "volume knob" turned too low or as signals in the brain not "gating" properly (that is, the signals are slow or poorly synched).

The **craving** of sensation typically occurs as a side-effect of oversensitivity or undersensitivity. Such craving is the incessant seeking of certain types of calming input that feel good (due to oversensitivity) or the constant attempt to experience sensation (due to undersensitivity). Commonly, we see children touching people or things, seeking out music or visual input, or sniffing things. Some children crave movement and their hyperactive behavior can be mistaken for ADHD.

Children with Autism and SMD

Children with ASD appear to have additional underlying causes of sensory sensitivity. Current research is focusing on "noisy" brain waves, lack of dendritic pruning, the connectivity between brain areas and the thickness of those connections. Some researchers note a general problem of signal bleed-over between sensory regions in the brain—both sub-cortical to cortical—and between individual sensory cortexes (such as visual and auditory).

Common problems for children with ASD include oversensitivity to smell, taste, sound and touch. Activities such as combing hair or clipping nails can register on the child's pain scale.

To get a sense of the problems children face, as well as the degree to which the problems linger through the years, let's look at some symptoms of poor sensory modulation. The example below describes the experiences of seven adults who have just arrived for a community meeting at city hall. Each person has a small or large modulation problem. Although each is now able to stay regulated in a social environment, they all had more serious issues as children.

- **Marcus** enters the room first and turns on all the lights: the fluorescents, the chandeliers and the spots. He then takes a seat and checks his email. He doesn't hear his friend, Ali, say hello to him from the doorway. Marcus is undersensitive to both sound and light. He is also a very picky eater and has symptoms of autism disorder spectrum, but not severe enough to have been diagnosed.

- **Esther** walks into the brightly lit room, shields her eyes and thinks, "Whew! This room's bright enough to do brain surgery in." She is sensitive to light. As a child, she used to scream when her sister turned on lights. Now she notices it, but doesn't complain.

- **Erica** walks in talking loudly to her friend, Miguel. Erica has a loud voice that often irritates her coworkers, and she is undersensitive to its volume. Erica chatters constantly and, in fact, she does so compulsively; she craves talking.

- **Jon** sits off to the far side. He is wearing a new silk shirt that feels luxurious to him. But the tags in the shirt are another matter. He had to cut them out prior to putting on the shirt. He is carrying a loosely woven, thick cotton sweater, and he plays with it nonchalantly, wrapping it around his hands to feel the texture with his fingers as he settles into his seat. As a child, he cringed when others touched him. As an adult, he is still sensitive to being touched, but doesn't react overtly to it. Although he is sensitive to touch and loves to touch soft textures, he is not overly sensitive to sound and doesn't even notice how loudly Erica is talking.

- Jon's wife, **Tania,** fidgets as she sits next to him. She has high energy and is constantly in motion. As a small child, her parents wondered if she had ADHD. She does, but she also has SMD, and she craves the sensation of movement.

- **Andrew,** wearing dark glasses, takes a seat in the back away from everyone else. He appears nervous. He had SMD as a child and continues to experience its symptoms as an adult. He doesn't like to be touched, and he doesn't tolerate light, loud noises (especially Erica's high-pitched voice) or smells. He noticed the scent of perfume as he entered and he is now obsessing on it. His thoughts tend to be disjointed and in a loop: "I asked the principal to send out a reminder telling people not to wear scent tonight. It's not right. They asked me to come. They should be considerate. I should leave."

- **Miguel,** a big easy-going man, slouches in his chair, crossing his arms and legs so they don't sprawl. He observes Andrew's dark glasses and nervous behavior and wonders about it. As a child, Miguel was undersensitive to sound and to sensations from his body. As a result, he had poor attention skills at school, and he was sedentary and somewhat overweight. He continues to have those issues, although coffee helps him to attend. He was diagnosed with the inattentive form of ADHD, but medication didn't change his symptoms. He doesn't have ADHD. He has SMD.

Through the years everyone in this group has learned strategies to compensate for their poor sensory modulation. As children mature into adulthood, most learn to tune out irritants and to tone down reactivity. However, some continue to struggle with unobtrusive symptoms that compromise their ability to function in normal environments and social settings.

The 'Upside' of SMD

There is an "upside" to having SMD symptoms. The child with oversensitivity might find nature, art, music, and touch to be exquisitely delightful as long as he is able to regulate the input. Alternatively, the person who craves sensory input has built-in motivation for learning a craft, art or skill that can provide that input. Craving might give the child the discipline to become a good musician, cook or runner. The child with undersensitivity is less disturbed by environmental factors than others, which sometimes produces an easy-going, laid-back personality.

Interoception

A common oversight is to restrict the conversation about sensory modulation to the five external senses, or to those five plus body movement and balance. There are additional internal senses (pain and temperature, for example) where modulation can be problematic for children with autism and other special needs. See the table for the traditional list of internal senses.

External senses	Internal senses
• Vision	• Temperature, pain, itch
• Hearing	• Vestibular (balance)
• Taste	• Proprioception (sense of body)
• Smell	• Hunger, thirst
• Touch	• Voiding

Another Look at Processing and Modulation

Let's revisit the process of registering, processing and acting upon sensory input. This time we will go further into the sensory-modulation circuitry.

Processing sensory data starts with the actual sensor (the eye, for example), which gathers light and color. That data is sent via nerves to the brain stem, up through the midbrain via thalamic tracts and into specialized cortical regions of the brain which attend to the raw input, identify it, and eventually store it in the sense's memory. As a part of that process, input from left and right sensors (for example, sound from both ears) cross to opposite sides of the brain via special tracts and the corpus callosum and then are integrated. Each sensory cortex performs initial identification of what it has received and then shares its findings with other relevant senses (e.g., vision shares with auditory) in the association cortex regions (the regions that integrate different types of input). If the sensory input was unusual or noteworthy, it is routed, along with cognitive and emotional data, to the cause-and-effect region of the brain: the right anterior insula (rAI) and the anterior cingulate cortex (ACC). The rAI decides what the brain should attend to, while the ACC triggers actions to take. Internal states such as hunger and body temperature are also monitored and acted on. Strong sensory input causes actions to be taken:

- It's too bright → put sunglasses on.
- I feel hunger → go find food and eat.

Not all strong input is attended to. The sun may be hurting my eyes, but other senses, cognitive states, or emotional states may contend for and win attention from the rAI. Resultant actions are typically motor or inhibitions of motor. Even sensation of felt emotions might cause motor changes to the face and gut. Actions might alter cognitive states, as well.

Here is an example of the decision-making process:

Jon is sensitive to sound, and his little sister likes to provoke him. She opens his bedroom door and blasts loud music to get a reaction. The loud volume is reported to Jon's rAI and selected for importance. A moment later, his rAI also notes strong feelings of irritation, as well as cognitive information informing him that he's seen this pattern of behavior from his sister many times before. The rAI attends to all of this and sends a decision to act to the ACC. Possible actions include:

- Jon could scream and slam the door
- He could inhibit those actions and quietly close the door
- He could glare at his sister with no reaction at all
- He could make a plan for revenge

In previous months, the noise would have triggered his scream. But he has been working on staying calm. As the sensory input arrives in the rAI, it is tempered by cognitive input reminding him not to react. He makes a decision to inhibit reacting. His ACC delivers motor commands to leave face muscles unchanged. He is proud of himself for not reacting, and now his emotional state adds weight to the decision. He decides to ignore her. His ACC delivers motor commands to quietly close the door.

The combined rAI and ACC are the final component in sensory modulation for all three types of symptoms (oversensitivity, undersensitivity and craving). They give us the opportunity to modify our behavior rather than to react to noxious sensory input, cave in to cravings or zone out due to low sensory registration. The combined rAI and ACC allow us to learn habits that will inspire a better response to the environment.

As with understanding the causes of SMD, we are still in the early stages of finding which strategies and interventions are effective. Many strategies and interventions have been found to be helpful to the child with sensory modulation disorder, and they are included in my book, *Self-Regulation Interventions and Strategies.* Here is a fairly exhaustive list of approaches you could take when working with a child. We'll look next at intervention effectiveness.

1. Try to eliminate the noxious input in the environment.
2. Give her greater control over her environment so that she can independently reduce the "volume" of the sensory input.
3. Try to block the input from her sensors (ears, eyes, mouth, nose, skin).
4. Try enriching the environment so that she is exposed to new, but pleasant sensation.
5. Mask unpleasant sensation with pleasant sensation.
6. Gradually expose her to a variety of input so that fewer sensations are "noteworthy" and cause a reaction.
7. Use desensitization techniques to help with acceptance of unpleasant input.
8. Train her in stress reduction so that her response to unpleasant input is moderated.
9. Train her to focus her attention on something else when there is unpleasant input, hoping that with time she will learn to ignore unpleasant sensation.
10. Train her in cognitive strategies and self-talk she can use within the rAI to help temper the response.
11. Educate her on the upsides of having SMD, and help her find ways to use her special set of sensitivity skills.
12. Immerse her in pleasant sensory input so she can relax and find joy.

The list is a mixture of approaches, strategies and interventions. Many approaches have been tried, but not many have been validated with rigorous study. The general approach that appears to work is exposure to sensory input. There are several classes of interventions within the exposure approach. Two types in this class are gradual exposure and desensitization, and both appear to work well. The evidence comes primarily from single case studies and small studies and shows good effect. For example, Koegel, et al (2012) demonstrated a therapeutic effect using exposure techniques in the area of feeding to overcome smell and taste sensitivities.

Another approach with good evidence is the sensory treatment developed by Jean Ayers, now known as Ayres Sensory Integration®. A review by Watling (2015) showed it is an effective treatment for sensory processing issues including some forms of sensory modulation. The Ayers technique primarily covers movement as well as visual and touch processing. Therapists trained in the method also learn to extrapolate the technique to functional areas such as feeding and toilet training when the underlying issues are sensory related. For example, Bellefeuille (2013) describes therapy using touch desensitization to enable successful toilet training.

A protocol-based exposure technique called Environmental Enrichment (described in chapters 3-5) has been shown to be effective in two studies. In this method, the child with autism is gradually alerted to simultaneous sensory input to two or more senses. The child's brain eventually learns to identify multiple streams of input, as well as to integrate data from multiple senses.

Sensory immersion, another exposure technique described in this book, promotes leisure skill development that can provide calming, pleasure and well-being. In this method, therapists and teachers use their knowledge of a child's sensory makeup to develop new sensory-based leisure skills in the child. The technique brings to life the adage "when life gives you lemons, make lemonade." The child learns to develop the gifts of her sensory differences and uses newly developed skills to help cope with sensory difficulties. Sensory immersion has not been studied as an independent intervention for sensory modulation. However, new research could be designed using methods and procedures, along with the detailed results of a study by Ismael (2015) who found correlations between children's sensory makeup and their leisure preferences and participation patterns.

Other popular exposure techniques such as listening therapy and the sensory diet have been written up in informal case studies, though they have not been formally studied for effectiveness.

A Continuum of Sensory Activities

This book uses exposure to sensory input as the primary intervention and presents a continuum of activities starting from the Environmental Enrichment protocol (chapters 3-5) to desensitization techniques (chapters 6, 7 and 8) to immersion activities that increase quality of life, quell cravings, and provide practice to undersensitive circuits (chapters 6-11).

Comparing Approaches that Can be Done without Special Equipment

As described above, there are many ways to provide sensory interventions. In this next section, we compare three exposure methods: sensory diets, sensory enrichment and the Environmental Enrichment protocol. Each of these can be done outside of the sensory clinic (that is, in a setting that does not have the special equipment found in a sensory gym). Following a brief description of each, we look at factors such as focus of the intervention and ease of implementation.

The **Environmental Enrichment program** is a formal protocol developed to provide a wide variety of sensory input twice daily to children with autism. The program increases awareness and tolerance of sensory input and helps the senses to integrate and work together. The program can be implemented at home, at school or within the context of an early intervention program.

Sensory enrichment interventions are put together as informal programs of graded sensory input as a way of helping the child to register certain types of input such as sound or touch to increase tolerance of them. The interventions are part of the standard practice of a school-based or clinic-based occupational therapist whose typical goal is to increase sensory awareness for the purpose of improved attention and behavior in the classroom.

Additionally, sensory immersion activities are provided to stimulate pleasurable sensory experiences, helping the child to relax and gain a sense of well-being.

Sensory diets are short motor-and-sensory exercise regimes that children perform throughout the day. The exercises are chosen based on the child's needs. The goal is increased regulation.

Comparing the Three Approaches

In general, all three of these approaches work to decrease symptoms of sensory modulation which will, in turn, increase attention skills and reduce undesirable behaviors such as meltdowns. However, the methods are quite different: they focus on different problems, and they challenge children in different ways. More important, some of them place difficult demands on the caregiver or teacher.

Environmental Enrichment (EE) exercises focus on ever-present sensory input like smells, sound and touch. Their goal is to bring the child's attention to the environment and register input. The exercises are sometimes passive and, as a group, are less challenging than sensory enrichment exercises. The protocol stipulates two 20-30 minute periods for enrichment activities, plus optional scent and sound immersion activities.

At the other end of the exercise spectrum, the sensory diet (SD) focuses on self-regulation throughout the day. It makes heavy use of motor activities that can help expend energy and calm the child. A sensory therapist identifies a number of sensorimotor activities that fit the child's needs and abilities. Every 90-120 minutes, the child's teacher or parent selects 10-15 minutes of activities from the therapist's set for the child to perform.

A sensory enrichment (SE) approach uses some of the same goals and types of interventions as the other two programs, but it is a flexible approach without a specified protocol. It covers a variety of intervention types. A sensory therapist selects activities, as well as duration and frequency of intervention, based on the child's need for registration of input or sensory desensitization or immersion. Parents and teachers are given supplemental home/classroom exercises. Sensory enrichment can be used as a source of substitute activities for the other programs.

The table below lays out the differences among the three programs in terms of target population (children with or without autism), ease of implementation, flexibility, commitment from parents and teachers, and level of evidence.

	Environmental Enrichment	**Sensory Enrichment**	**Sensory Diet**
Target Population	ASD	Sensory or ASD	Sensory or ASD
Goals	Increase attention to environment. Acclimate to environment. Reduce behaviors.	Gradually increase child's ability to modulate in the presence of sensory input.	Train child's brain and body to stay regulated. Decrease feeling of being overwhelmed.
Focus on specific sense	Many are covered, but primary focus is on combined scent and touch, sound, light touch and thermal.	Focus is on the child's most problematic sensory areas.	Focus on movement strategies to provide calming, as well as input to other senses as needed.
Ease of implementation	Purchase materials and follow the protocol.	Select activities based on child's needs and interests. Exercises can be incorporated into daily activities.	Therapist determines child's sensory needs and finds suitable exercises. Caregivers select activities from a list.
Number of interventions per day	Two 20-30 minute semi-structured sessions. Optionally, two 1-minute scent immersion and a 15-minute music immersion.	Not prescribed. 2-3 times per week, minimum.	One 1—15 minute session every 90-120 minutes throughout the day.
Flexibility	Somewhat flexible. Set procedure, but flexible times.	Very flexible.	Flexible activities but set times.
Compliance	Somewhat demanding. Parents and teachers need to be well organized.	Not structured. Caregivers and teachers may forget to perform activities.	In an unstructured environment, parents and teachers find compliance to be difficult.
Evidence	Two studies show evidence with children with autism. Many animal model studies.	Not studied as a stand-alone technique, but commonly integrated in effective feeding and Ayers Sensory Integration® techniques.	Not sufficiently studied as a stand-alone technique. It is a component of Therapressure™ which has a "Level 2" evidence rating.

A Note About Screening and Assessment Tools

A number of sensory modulation screening tools are currently on the market, and a new assessment (the Sensory Scales) is in trial. Sensory therapists typically screen with the Sensory Profile (SP), the Short Sensory Profile (SSP) or the Sensory Processing Measure (SPM). All three are parent and teacher questionnaires and are standardized and normed. As screening tools, they work well at identifying problem areas of SMD and related behavioral issues. However, they do not identify underlying issues in the sensory system. A side note: the SSP and SP are typically used by researchers to categorize the sensory makeup of their study population.

(A free informal checklist is available on the SPD Foundation website at http://www.spdfoundation. net/about-sensory-processing-disorder/symptoms/. This set of questions is not standardized or normed, but provides a starting point for determining sensory-modulation issues.)

Programs and Practice

When it comes to changing the way the body operates, OTs and PTs believe in exercise with lots of practice. Sensory therapists also agree that, in order to increase sensory processing and modulation skills, the child needs a regular program of activities. They can be loose or highly structured, yet they should be reasonably consistent. The challenge is to determine the optimum number of interventions in a day or a week. The standard practice for OTs and PTs consists of two in-clinic (or in-school) sessions per week with assigned at-home activities. The Environmental Enrichment protocol mandates two 15-30 minute exercise blocks each day. That was too much for 25 percent of the parents who dropped out of the study due to time constraints. (The remaining parents managed to facilitate their child's program about 77 percent of the time, which was sufficient to produce significant results.) The Star Center, a sensory clinic in Denver, uses an intensive model with month-long, on-site treatment. They have reported excellent results.

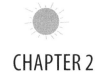

CHAPTER 2

Working with Children

This chapter describes in detail a systematic approach for working (and playing) with children with sensory processing disorder, including SMD. This includes most children with autism and some with ADHD. This chapter is based on the work of leading sensory researchers who named **10 core elements** for providing effective sensory interventions for children (Parnham, 2007).

Practices have evolved in the ensuing years since the researchers identified these core elements, but these guiding principles remain a good foundation for practice. This chapter includes "best practices" for a clinic setting that can be used, as well, in school settings and at home. Guidance for parent and classroom involvement has been woven into these recommendations to assist parents and teachers who are working on their own with children.

The "Core Elements"

Here is a list of the core elements.

1. Create opportunities for the child to gain sensory (or executive function or social or emotional) experiences.
2. Collaborate with the child.
3. Give the child "just the right challenge."
4. Gently guide the child through the process of making choices and plans.
5. Help the child to maintain a calm-alert state.
6. Make therapy activities fun and engaging.
7. Modify activities to ensure the child's success.
8. Keep the child physically safe.
9. Set-up the environment to motivate the child.
10. Create a strong rapport with the child.

These elements form a set of guidelines for those who wish to incorporate sensory practices into their work with children. This next section explains each of the elements and gives advice on how to make use of them in practice.

1. Create opportunities for experience

The goal is to provide children various experiences in the areas of sensory processing, executive function, social growth and emotional awareness. Let's begin with sensory activities. The following two statements are true: 1) sensory interventions do not need to be done as a stand-alone activity, and 2) any activity can become a sensory activity. Now replace the word *sensory* with the other types of activities: executive function, social growth and emotional awareness, and read the two statements again. They remain true. If you can find ways to add sensory (or executive function, social growth and emotional awareness) into the day's planned activities, you can add value (i.e., achieve sensory goals) with just a little extra work.

Most of the activities in this book are focused on sensory and sensory-motor, and they are typically performed with children with sensory needs. So let's dig down deeper and discuss ways we can create opportunities for sensory interventions.

Create opportunities for sensory experience

Although parents and educators can perform a sensory-only activity such as having a child smell a vial of scent or listen to calming music, the mixing of sensory into normal day-to-day activities saves time and supports overall growth and development. In therapy, combining sensory with another intervention makes for a richer, potentially more powerful intervention. The challenge is to create a sensory mindset. You can incorporate sensory with other activities in the following ways:

- Keep on hand materials like those suggested in the list below.
- Approach each task with the question: what can I add to this activity to make it more pleasant or more challenging?
- Play your strong suit. Find the easiest way for you to work with the child: arts and crafts, motor activities, games, stories, puppets, academic work, play activities, cooking, housework or something else. Start with one activity and add a single extra sensory component. For example, use scented crayons with a coloring-book activity. Add punching pillows (proprioceptive input) to the task of making the bed. Add singing songs to performing chores or to playing with puppets. Take shoes off for a little while when taking a walk.

When we combine sensory input with the other things we are doing, integration of the senses with the brain and body takes place.

Have these on hand:

1. Natural scents to sniff or to add to activity materials (3-4 of these):
   a. Jars of orange peel, lemon peel, dried mint, fennel seed or anise seed (licorice);
   b. A bottle of real vanilla;
   c. Diluted essential oils: a few drops of real fruit or flower scents in a small jar of water (check for allergens before using flowers).

2. Music player, calming music, speakers and headphones.

3. Visual:
   a. Coloring materials (design coloring books for older children);
   b. A kaleidoscope;
   c. Colorful magazines.

4. Fidgets (get a few of these):
   a. Two feet (2/3 m.) of Thera-Tube or Thera-Band (OT or PT will have these);
   b. A personal container of Thera-Putty for each child;
   c. Velcro with adhesive backing to put on bottom edge of a table (for rubbing finger tips on);
   d. 2 sandbags covered with colorful material– to fit into the hand;
   e. Soft materials, toys for feeling and squeezing.

5. Regulating items (1 or more of these):
   a. Weighted balls: 1-2 pounds (.5-1 kilo) for 2-year-olds. 5 pounds (2 kilos) for 8-year-olds, 8-12 pounds (4-5 kilos) for older children;
   b. A body sock or stretchy fabric tubing for deep pressure play (find these online);
   c. A rocking chair;
   d. Sugarless gum, mints, sour candies.

6. Vibration:
   a. Pillow or stuffed animal;
   b. Electric toothbrush (at home).

2. Collaborate with the child

Collaboration with an older child on plans and activities for a session, as well as child-directed play with a younger child, is a win-win for all. The child feels respected and gets a sense of control and ownership in the interventions. For the therapist, teacher or parent, the interactive sessions can be fun as well as effective.

Child-directed play is *not* a free-for-all with the child now running amok. Instead, the therapist suggests activities and observes the child as she plays, looking for opportunities to incorporate lessons and introduce challenges. The therapist ensures that the child is keeping pace with the work and that the child is engaged by adjusting the level of stimulation (through lighting and sound). The therapist also grades the emotional intensity and other factors by introducing calming or alerting activities.

Every therapist, teacher or parent brings their own personality and style to collaboration. One person might collaborate using a matter-of-fact negotiation technique. Another might be quite playful, but have a solid plan in mind. Let's look at two scenarios.

Scenario 1: Roger is a matter-of-fact sort of therapist. Prior to seeing a child, he creates a plan with goals. On the day of the session, he puts together engaging activities, sets out interesting materials and asks the child to do the work. On a good day, the child comes in, looks to see what Roger has in store for him and does his work. Another day, the child may enter and complain about the activity. Roger listens, collaborates, negotiates and works with the child. If they can compromise, the child happily completes the work. However, the child may have his own agenda that day. In that case, Roger can elect to take it easy, gently incorporating elements that will accomplish his (Roger's) goals. If the child is resistant on a regular basis, Roger can use behavioral methods to rein him in.

Scenario 2: Fiona is seeing a small child with autism, and she uses a picture schedule to help him track activities. Although she knows what she wants to do before he arrives, she waits for him before setting up the schedule. After he arrives she enlists his help in selecting the activities by showing him three cards and asking, "Which of these should we do?" Next, she gets his input in choosing the order in which they'll be done by asking, "*This* first, or *this* first?" In giving the child control over small decisions, Fiona gets better compliance.

3. Give the child just-the-right challenge

Perhaps the best known of the ten core elements is "Give the child the just-right challenge." How can we tell how much input a child needs? This can be tricky. While we want to provide a child with challenge, we need to keep challenges appropriate to her intellect, sensory systems, attention skills, emotional system and physical body. The best way to do so is to tune in to the child as you work with her. Sense her calm-alert state, her frustration level, her attention-to-task and her capacity for enjoyment. Later, get feedback from the child, as well as from caregivers and teachers on how well she was able to handle the remainder of the day.

Two important observations:

- In terms of sensory stimulation, the child's environment should have just the right amount of sensory stimulus. The sensory-sensitive child and the child with autism might show subtle reactions to loud noises, bright lights and to being touched. You need to address these environmental factors. The undersensitive child may need stronger sensory input such as lively music or physical exercise to wake up sleepy circuits in the brain. The child who craves input such as touch or enjoys visual "stimming" may need a specific amount of that input from time to time to satisfy the craving and allow self-regulation. Giving that child a two-minute break to receive the sensory input he craves will help him to attend.

- The child with ADHD may have a limited supply of brain glucose, the substance that provides energy to brain self-regulation circuits (in the prefrontal cortex). He may be able to perform, for example, the attention-to-task activities that you give him, but doing so depletes his store of brain glucose. That will limit his ability to self-regulate once he leaves you, and he might act out with impulsivity or other behaviors immediately afterwards. The just-right challenge will consider his capacity to switch gears and stay regulated after your session. It might include hard work with a rest period and protein snack (such as a glucose shake) immediately afterward. (Glucose shakes are available over the counter at pharmacies. Check with parents and the child's doctor beforehand.)

4. Guide the child through the process of making choices and plans

Many interventions with children with autism, ADHD and sensory disorders include an education component. Children getting sensory interventions learn (in a hands-on method) about the level of sensory input their brain needs and can tolerate. A child with ADHD will learn tricks to pay better attention and to monitor his own level of impulsivity and hyperactivity. The child with autism also learns these things, plus how to express and read emotions, how to communicate with others, and how to use simple organization techniques such as a visual schedule. When we teach children through role-play or other forms of live simulation, we have the opportunity to include some self-reflection. Using a cognitive approach, we can interject open questions such as, "How did that feel?" and "What would you do in this situation?" and "How do you know when you've reached your limit?" We can also ask leading questions throughout the intervention that will help him to understand the process, for instance, "What should we do next?" "Is this a good idea or a bad idea?" "What will happen if we . . .?"

In the same way, we can interject questions such as, "Which goes first?" or "What do we do next?" Other questions can walk the child through decision-making, organization and planning out an activity.

5. Help the child to maintain a calm-alert state

Not all worthwhile activities call for a calm-alert state, yet it is the best state for learning and participating. There are a number of ways to calm a child and to increase her level of alertness.

Physical activities help provide a calm-alert state. They include heavy work, chores, exercises, aerobics, sports, swimming and so on. On-the-spot calming from excitement can be achieved with a 4-minute workout (see chapter 10). Gentle movement, rocking, and swaying are calming. Fast movement and dancing are alerting. Some children become overactive with movement and need a calming exercise afterwards. Playing toss with a heavy ball can calm an excited child within a minute or two.

Sensory activities include adjustment of lighting and sound – up for alerting, down for calming. Cold, tangy, minty or spicy foods and drinks are alerting. Warm foods and drinks, as well as mushy foods, are calming. Root vegetables (potatoes, beets, yams, carrots) and mushrooms are thought to be calming. Turkey is known for its soporific effect. Bright, fast music is alerting; soft slow music is calming. The sound and activity of a group will be alerting and may decrease a child's ability to be calm. Working solo may decrease alertness but is calmer.

We can adjust a child's calm and alert states by the activities we choose. Calming activities are generally slower and rhythmic and may involve slow breathing or singing. Alerting activities can include physical movement, singing or reciting. We can grade the activity level (the intensity of the activity) to match the needs of the child. Citrus or vanilla scent in small quantities can also help provide a calm-alert state (see chapter 7: scent immersion).

When working with a new child with autism, ADHD or sensory disorders, it's important to build the start of a relationship by doing fun or interesting activities for a few minutes. Have the child do a few minutes of movement prior to asking him to sit and work. Movement helps get wiggles out of the body and increases focus for work.

Movement gives you a chance to tune-in to his energy level, personality and various cues or signals concerning his state of mind and emotions. Look also for other signals, such as eyes that squint at bright light (demonstrating light sensitivity), a body that becomes stiff in a noisy environment, darting eyes showing inattention, silly behaviors that reveal underlying emotions, and so on.

Prior to a difficult activity such as feeding therapy, socialization or sensory desensitization, have the child do 15 to 20 minutes of strenuous play or work. This helps ground the child and makes him less resistant to the task. Activities that make use of the upper body and that get the child breathing hard help to relax the shoulder and neck muscles that easily become tense with anxiety. Such activities include climbing, hanging from a trapeze or monkey bars, or doing wall push-ups, floor push-ups or chair push-ups.

A child ready to have a meltdown will reveal cues through body language. You might see rounded shoulders, a sad demeanor and eyes that look at the floor. Or you might see an arched back and arms and legs spread open and ready to flail.

A therapist, teacher or parent who disregards subtle (or not-so-subtle) signs of discontent in a child with autism, ADHD or sensory disorders may have to deal with a volatile situation. The child's mood has not been acknowledged, and now he might act-out in frustration to gain attention. A simple statement such as, "You look upset," can help to avoid undesirable behaviors. If the child is verbal, a small discussion is appropriate if he is willing to talk. Otherwise, setting him up in a quiet environment with quiet activities can help him transition to a better mood.

A child who is having a meltdown benefits from being in a low-lit, quiet room. Soft, soothing speech from you, along with slow movement in a rocking chair, swing or swaying in your arms, can be helpful. Some children accept hugs, others do not. Take things slowly if you do not know the child well. It takes a bit of time to recover from a strong mood or an emotional outburst, and modification of the child's activities and our expectations of her may be needed.

In other cases, a few minutes of quiet activity is enough for the child to calm. If we gradually increase the pace of activity, along with the beat of background music and the brightness of the room, the child can be transitioned to normal activities.

6. Make the activities fun and engaging

Look for ways to turn mundane tasks into creative learning experiences that engage the child. There are many ways of accomplishing tasks. For example, a child can be taught multiplication tables by writing them out on paper four times each, or she could recite them while clapping and stamping her feet in rhythm to a beat, or she could sing them very softly to a gentle tune. The goal has been met each time, but the means are completely different – and some of the means are fun. Which do we choose? If they appear to be equally effective, why not choose the fun option.

7. Modify activities to ensure the child's success

It goes without saying that we need to modify or grade activities that are too challenging for a child. Think about the child's physical, sensory, mental, self-regulatory, emotional and social limitations. If we ask a child with ADHD to sit quietly for a long period and perform work she does not want to do, we risk her chances for success. Likewise, asking a boy with high functioning autism to participate in a noisy group activity with interactive discussion might cause him to be anxious and to act out. We can make both these scenarios work if we grade the level of challenge. In the first case, modifying the length of the task or using a more interesting activity (or both) will increase her ability to succeed. In the second, we can modify the goal such that he is expected to tolerate a group function for all or part of its duration, but he is not (yet) expected to participate in the discussion.

We can increase the child's chances for success in other ways as well by following the advice of Dr. Lucy Miller, head of the STAR Center in Denver. Families travel to the center for a month-long intensive therapy treatment for their child with sensory processing disorder (with or without autism). The child receives several therapy sessions each day during the month. This intensive schedule increases the child's skills dramatically in a short amount of time. Parents are included in the sessions. This allows parents to "share in the success," as well as to learn new ways to be with their child and to help him maintain his new-found skills when they return home.

Based on this model, consider including others (teachers, parents, aides and other therapists) in your treatments, so that the child receives successful therapy that can be carried over to other environments by those who participated in it.

8. Keep the child physically safe

Safety is always an important concern, and adults are generally aware of safety hazards such as small or sharp items, trip hazards, and safety issues associated with play equipment. Additional concerns are involved in working with children with autism, ADHD and sensory processing disorders. A few of the common safety risks are listed below.

- Children who crave sensory input might take unwarranted risks by chewing on unsafe items, jumping from high places, listening to loud music over headphones, touching things and people at random, and so on.

- A child who is undersensitive to temperature or pain might scald himself while running water or a bath, or hurt himself without realizing it.

- Children who are undersensitive to their body movement (vestibular and proprioceptive senses), as well as children with ADHD, are at higher risk than others for injury and accidents during play. Such a child might also underestimate his strength as he plays with another child.

- A child who is oversensitive to touch or sound or is poorly regulated overall might lash out at others and cause them harm.

It is also important, of course, to keep the child emotionally safe. When you know your client or student well, you understand what types of things might trigger a strong emotional reaction. Common triggers include loud sounds, touching, removal of a favorite object, separation anxiety from parents, frustration in not being able to perform a task, lack of control, and so on.

9. Set up the environment to motivate the child

Setting up the work and play space is key to a good intervention. The space needs to be simple enough that the child is not overwhelmed by the choices of play. Yet it needs to suggest that play opportunities are available. In one version of an ideal setting, two games might be sitting on a table, a swing is available, a drum is sitting in a corner and, in a clinic, a trampoline is set up. These props guide children in activity, giving them choices of equally suited activities or suggesting rewards for non-preferred work.

You can modify the sensory elements of the environment using the standard elements of light (soft for quiet, bright for alert), music (soft or loud, fast or slow), and even put natural scent in the room to increase a sense of comfort. These elements support the child's sensory systems and, in turn, his emotional state and may prevent a downward or upward spiral.

10. Create a strong rapport with the client

Create a rapport with the child that will motivate her to accept challenges and to work hard during interventions. Every therapist, educator or parent has their own style for being and working with children. Some are playful, some are more directive. It's best to try to include aspects of both playfulness and no-nonsense structure in your interactions with children. A pleasant demeanor and a playful attitude can go a long way toward getting the child to bond with you. Establishing rules and setting boundaries help to ensure that activities do not get out of control and create friction. Shared activities like games, role playing, puppets, and races can be shared fun that help the child to engage and bond. Finally, remember that you are asking the child to work hard, so make sure that you reward her for her efforts with preferred or fun activities.

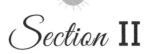

Section II

THE ENVIRONMENTAL ENRICHMENT PROTOCOL

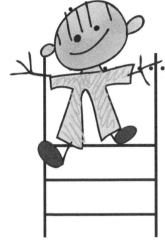

This section contains a guide for implementing the Environmental Enrichment protocol. Included are specific instructions for performing the protocol activities, a list of needed materials and the details for performing each of the protocol's 34 enrichment exercises.

The Environmental Enrichment protocol for children with autism spectrum disorder (ASD) is a six-month multi-sensory exposure program whose goal is to stimulate children's senses and increase sensory processing skills. The program was designed to be a low-cost way for parents of children with autism to personally provide effective treatment in a home setting. However, as described below, other settings will work when supplemented by home-based activities.

In this program, children perform a graduated series of exercises during two 15-30 minute work periods. The exercises provide input to two or more senses simultaneously. The primary sources for sensory input are scent, touch, sound, vision, thermal (hot/cold), and vestibular (balance). The activities are relatively straightforward: sniff this, put feet in hot water, walk on this board, and so on. Materials needed for the activities are readily found in the home or community.

The protocol is based on methods of sensory enrichment found to work effectively in autism animal models. A protocol was designed for children and tested. Following successful case studies, two controlled studies were conducted (Woo and Leon, 2013; Woo, Donnelly, Steinberg-Epstein & Leon, 2015).

Twenty-eight children ages 3-12 took part in the first study. Half of the children received standard care which was defined to be: Applied Behavior Therapy (ABA), occupational therapy, speech therapy, social skills training and adapted physical therapy. The other half received standard care and the enrichment protocol. At the end of six months, children in the enrichment protocol group showed a decrease in severity of autism symptoms using the Childhood Autism Rating Scale (CARS), as well as an increase in cognition and receptive language. (There was no change in expressive language and sensory symptoms were not assessed.) These results were strong and were independent of the child's age.

In the 2015 study, 91 children ages 3-6 were recruited, matched for age and symptom severity and divided into three groups: A control group receiving standard care, a full-protocol group (as in the first study) and a partial-protocol group that used a reduced version of the protocol. There was high attrition overall due to a variety of factors and only 50 children completed the study. The results were again significant. Children in the enrichment groups showed a decrease in severity of autism symptoms (using the Autism Diagnostic Observation Schedule, or ADOS) over their peers who received standard care. A surprising result was that one in five children in the enrichment groups no longer qualified for the autism label (p=.01). There was an increase in cognition, receptive language, and a decrease in sensory issues (as assessed by the Short Sensory Profile.) The study showed a "medium-size" effect which was independent of age. The research teams concluded that the protocol is a low-cost, effective treatment for children with ASD. One last finding to note: the researchers looked for factors that correlated losing the label and found that those children who did had higher combined cognition and language skills scores than their peers. A higher cognitive score or language skill score alone did not increase the likelihood of losing the label.

Getting Started with the Environmental Enrichment Protocol

The environmental enrichment program was designed to keep costs low, and so it is meant to be done without the support of an occupational therapist or other sensory therapist. However, it does help to think like a sensory therapist when implementing the protocol. This book contains a great deal of supplementary material to help you do just that.

Prior to getting started:

1. Read chapter 2, *Working with Children*, which presents a sensory therapist's framework for performing sensory interventions with children.

2. Browse through the exercises in chapter 4 and familiarize yourself with the format. Note that chapter 4 provides help to those implementing the protocol by:
   a) Providing thorough instructions for each exercise;
   b) Grading each exercise with easier and harder activities;
   c) Making the exercise content more interesting;
   d) Noting the safety and sensory considerations for each exercise;
   e) Listing the goals for each exercise;
   f) Suggesting methods for self-regulation techniques to calm or alert the child as he or she adapts to the rigors of the program.

3. Carefully read the instructions in chapter 3. They contain program implementation details and attempt to predict and solve many of the problems that might be encountered.

4. Browse through the "mix-ins" in chapter 4—speech, motor and rhythm activities—that can be done independently or alongside the protocol.

CHAPTER 3

Program Instructions

The Protocol

The protocol runs for six months. There are two versions, the short version and the long one, described in detail below. The short version has a simpler regimen and requires fewer materials. It can more easily be performed within the school (or early intervention) environment. The long version adds scents and music to the day and has a larger base of exercises to draw from. Objectively, the two regimens are similarly effective in terms of the gains seen in IQ and in the Autism Diagnostic Observation scores (ADOS). However, parents who completed the long version found that scents were helpful in providing increased regulation and calming to their child, and they would therefore do them again. Although the studies did not note any benefit from listening to classical music, music and music therapy have been shown to be helpful in reducing behaviors, and stimulating social skills in children with autism.

The Activities

The core of the program consists of two 15-30 minute enrichment sessions in which the child performs 4-7 activities. This section lists the exercises, describes the effort needed to perform them, and then discusses alternative exercises that were created for children of different abilities. The next chapter provides thorough details for performing all exercises.

The 34 exercises of the long version of the protocol are listed in the table below. The short version uses only 15 of these (**indicated in bold type in the table**).

Activity Number	Activity
1	**Place hands and feet in water of different temperatures**
2	**Squeeze objects of different shapes and textures**
3	**Draw imaginary lines on the child's face and arms**
4	**Walk on a pathway of different textures blindfolded**
5	**Draw lines on the child's face, arms, and legs with objects while listening to music**
6	**Find the twin of an object in a pillowcase**
7	Take a scented bath then get a massage with scented oil or scented lotion
8	While speaking or singing, touch arms and legs with a cooled or warmed spoon
9	**Draw lines on arms and legs with cooled or warmed spoons**
10	**Match a picture of an object to the real object**
11	**Walk on a 2 x 8-inch x 5-foot plank with eyes open, then blindfolded**
12	**Remove a colored bead from a dish filled with ice cubes**

Activity Number	Activity
13	**Use a sound cue to distract attention away from a visual task**
14	**Remove objects from bowls of cool and warm water**
15	**Pull a button from between someone's fingers**
16	Walk on a bouncy surface of foam or large pillow with eyes open, then blindfolded
17	**Point to objects in a picture and name them**
18	Place a finger on a cool object, then on a warm one
19	Create a small depression in dough and then put rice in it
20	Select a textured square that matches its photo
21	Draw imaginary circles on the child's face using textured objects
22	Place ice-filled straws into dough, alternating hands
23	Walk on a 2 x 8-inch x 5-foot plank while carrying a chilled tray
24	Rub fingers and toes in turn while child watches
25	Place coins in a piggy bank using only a mirrored reflection of hands
26	Pick up small objects using a thin pole with a magnet attached
27	Track a red object as it moves around a picture
28	Walk up and down stairs while holding a big ball or pillow
29	Draw shapes using pencil and paper to match the shapes being drawn on the child's back (over shirt)
30	Draw lines on paper using both hands simultaneously
31	**Match colored beads to the colors of objects in a photo**
32	Blow aluminum foil or a small feather on the floor as far as possible
33	View two pictures as they repeatedly move from back to front and back again
34	Listen to music that corresponds in subject matter to a photo

The activities are simple but the setup may take a bit of time. Let's look at the first activity: *Place hands and feet in water of different temperatures.* Assuming that containers such as bowls or pails have been obtained, setup for this exercise is simple. Fill the containers with water of different temperatures. Contrast that exercise with the fourth exercise in which the child walks on a pathway of different textures. The setup may entail moving furniture to make room for a walkway near a wall, and then creating the pathway.

The activities can be and should be adjusted for each child, depending on their age, functional skills and sensory skills. To that end, most activity descriptions (in the next chapter) have both easier and harder alternate activities to be done in place of the original activity. The activity also notes safety and sensory considerations and workarounds to problems.

Short version

Here is the short version of the protocol:

• Perform 4-7 prescribed multi-sensory activities (from a total set of 15 sensory activities) twice each day, separated by three or more hours, for 15-30 minutes at a time.

Time commitment: 40-75 minutes total daily for setup and facilitation of the two exercise periods.

Long version

Here is the long version of the protocol:

1. Listen to classical music for 15 minutes over headphones.
2. Smell natural scents while receiving a one-minute back rub 4 times a day.
3. Perform 4-7 prescribed multi-sensory activities (from the total set of 34 sensory exercises) twice each day for 15-30 minutes at a time.
4. Sleep with a scented cotton ball in the pillowcase.

Splitting up the work for the long version: There is a considerable time commitment in doing the long version of the protocol, but there is also a great deal of flexibility in how it gets done. Exercises can be done in the home by parents alone, or by a combination of parents, aides and therapists who come to the home. Likewise, they can be done during the week in a school or early intervention setting and in the home on weekends and holidays. Here are sample schedules for the child receiving the program entirely at home (top schedule) or in a combination of school and home.

Sample home schedule

Time	Activity
8:30–8:31 am	Scent and back rub
10:00-10:30 am	Exercises plus scent and back rub
2:00-2:30 pm	Exercises plus scent and back rub
5:30-5:31 pm	Scent and back rub
8:30-8:45 pm	Classical music
8:45 pm	Place scented cotton ball in pillow

Sample school/home schedule

Time	Activity	Facilitator
7:30–7:31 am	Scent and back rub	Parent
10:00-10:30 am	Exercises plus scent and back rub	School aide (Parent on weekends)
2:00-2:30 pm	Exercises plus scent and back rub	School aide (Parent on weekends)
5:30-5:31 pm	Scent and back rub	Parent
8:30-8:45 pm	Classical music	Parent
8:45 pm	Place scented cotton ball in pillow	Parent

To decrease the load, you can trim the two exercise sessions to 15-20 minutes instead of 15-30 minutes. You can also perform a scent and back rub activity immediately before or after the exercise sessions, and combine the music and last scent activity with the child's bedtime routine.

Should I do the short version or the long version?

Start with the short version. If you can add in scent one or more times per day, do that. Likewise, try to find time each day for calming music. Add additional exercises from the long version, as desired, for variety and to decrease the rigidity of the exercise schedule.

The Mix-ins

Following the 34 enrichment exercises (in chapter 4) are additional exercises to facilitate speech, gross motor, and rhythm and timing. The speech exercises are designed to encourage expressive communication. They include reading books together, playing simple instruments and doing activities that make noise. The motor exercises were selected to increase functional and novel movement, and to enhance the child's sense of motor rhythm.

Most of the mix-ins are fun and can be added into the exercise sessions as an interlude or offered at the end as a reward for completing the exercises. They do not replace the original set of exercises.

Program Instructions

Instructions are given for the long version. If you are doing the short version of the program, optionally skip the sections covering scent and music.

About the Exercises

Weeks 1 & 2: For the most part, the 34 exercises are ordered by difficulty. On the first day, start with exercises 1-5 just as they are. As you are doing them, informally assess the challenge of each exercise for the child. If one exercise is too hard, select one of the "easier activities" (at the end of that exercise) to do in place of the original. Likewise, if the activity is too easy, select a "harder" activity.

If you are not able to complete five exercises within the time period (i.e. 30 minutes), scale the number of exercises back to four. Alternately, if you complete all five and have time to do more, add one or two more. Perform this group of exercises for two weeks, using additional easier or harder activities as seems logical.

Weeks 3 & 4: Before adding the next set of exercises (e.g., numbers 6-10) to the regimen, you need to decide whether to continue with any of the current activities. Here are some general guidelines for making that decision:

- If the child struggled with the easier activities in the exercise and was not able to accomplish the base (original) exercise, continue with it. If he dislikes the exercise, don't force him to do it, but continue to expose him to those materials so that he becomes accustomed to them.

- If he seems to enjoy a particular activity, and there is nothing similar to it in the upcoming exercises, you can optionally continue working with it.

- If the child is tired of an exercise, but you think he needs to continue with it, drop it for now. (You can come back to it later.)

- Drop any exercise the child seems to have mastered unless you want to continue with some of the harder activities suggested at the end of that exercise. For example, if the child appears comfortable with playing in different temperatures of water (exercise 1), but upon looking at the harder exercises, you decide that he could benefit from some fine-motor play with warm and cool objects, then you might keep the first exercise or mark it and come back to later.

Once you have decided which exercises to keep, add additional ones to the child's regimen. The 34 exercises are generally graded by difficulty, and so the best plan is to do them in the order in which they are presented.

Additional weeks: Every two weeks, set up exercises for the next period following the rules given above for weeks 3 and 4. Eventually, all of the exercises will have been completed and you will need to repeat the ones done previously. Do not stop at that time, but continue the program for the full six months. Use one or more of the following methods to choose which activities to revisit during the remainder of the six-month period.

1. Continue to rotate in order through the 34 basic exercises for the six month period.

2. Select activities based on need. For instance, if the child is still struggling with balance, make sure that *walking with and without blindfold* exercises are in the mix.

3. Select activities that give the child a variety of different sensations.

4. Randomly select activities from the basic exercises, while making sure that there is variety within the group of them.

5. If the child is doing very well, you might try substituting similar activities from the sensory enrichment chapter (chapter 5).

Recurring themes in the activities

There are recurring themes graded by difficulty in the exercise sets. The lists below map the exercises by sensory element (hot/cold, touch, motor, visual, scent, and hearing) and by overall topic (play with cold items, manipulation control, naming objects, and so on). The numbers next to each topic are the exercise numbers that pertain to that topic. For example, visual matching can be found in exercises 10, 12, 20 and 31. Numbers in bold are exercises in the short version of the protocol. A few activities are listed in multiple categories.

You can make use of the lists as you select new activities by skipping ahead to a harder one if the current one is too simple. For example, if exercise 12 (motor, fine motor) is too simple, skip ahead to exercise 15. Likewise, you can fall back to an easier one (or to the easier activities) if the child is struggling.

Cold / Hot

- Hands, feet in bowls: **1, 14**
- Coolness /warmth on skin: 8, **9**, 18
- Play with cold items: **12**, 22
- Carry cooled item: 23

Touch

- Textured objects: **2,** 19, 20, 22
- Draw lines on skin + texture: **3, 5,** 21
- Matching objects with blindfold: 6
- Touch and fine motor: **15**, 25
- Massage: 24

Motor

- Walk path, blindfold, textures: **4, 11,** 16, 23
- Fine motor: **12, 15,** 19, 25, 26
- Climb stairs: 28
- Draw: 29, 30
- Blowing: 32

Visual

- Blindfold match, blindfold walk: **4, 6, 11**, 16
- Matching: **10, 12**, 20, **31**
- Attention and tracking: **13**, 27, 33
- Naming objects: **17**
- Visual-auditory: 34

Scent

- Bath scent, oil: 7
- Smell odorant 4 times a day
- Put scent in pillowcase every night

Hearing

- Visual-auditory: 34
- Distract from visual: **13**
- Listen to music once each day

Performing the Exercises

The exercises session is 15-30 minutes long. Have the child perform each activity in the session for three to five minutes. Try these suggestions to fill the time: repeat each exercise multiple times, vary an exercise by making little games as you do it, talk about the sensations he feels, name the objects used, and ask questions about his experience.

To help ensure you keep track of the three to five minute period, set a timer. A visual timer with a bell is best. Look to see if your phone or tablet has one. Optionally, download an app or purchase an egg timer. To help with transition from one exercise to the next, use a visual (picture) schedule. Each of the activities in this book has a picture associated with it that you can copy and use in the child's visual schedule. Better yet, make use of your phone or camera to make your own pictures.

It is important to do the exercises consistently both during the week and on weekends. However, good results were obtained by parents in the studies who completed the protocols 77% of the time. If a child is getting the protocol in school, arrangements should be made for parents to continue the work at home on weekends. In most cases, the materials and equipment needed are easy to find, so access to materials should not limit participation. However, in cases where certain activities are too difficult to perform in the child's home environment, the parent can substitute a complementary exercise. For example, if the child is scheduled to do exercise 6 (climbing stairs while holding a pillow), but stairs aren't available at home, think of an alternate way of doing it, such as stepping up and down off of a stool while holding a pillow.

Using scents

If you are doing the scent exercises, you will need seven odorants (scents) to work with. You will be preparing seven jars of odorants using essential oils, and you'll need seven clean vials or jars with caps, a bag of clean cotton balls and seven different (small) jars of essential oil. Woo and Leon used child-friendly scents including anise, apple, hibiscus, lemon, sweet orange, banana, and apricot. Prepare seven jars to hold the odorants in the following way: put a cotton ball into each empty vial, put 1 drop of essential oil on the cotton ball, and close the jar tightly. Label each jar with the odorant it contains (apple, sweet orange, and so on).

Four times during the day, expose the child to an odorant—each time using a different scent. To do this:

1. Open a jar of odorant and tell the child to breathe in the smell.

2. At the same time, gently rub the child's back with a fisted hand.

3. Continue doing this for one minute.

4. Reclose the jar tightly.

5. Add a drop of oil to the cotton ball whenever the scent begins to fade.

Rotate through the odorants in order. If the child finds a scent disagreeable, replace it with a different scent. Children are also exposed to a fragrance at night by placing a scented cotton ball in their pillowcase before bedtime. You can simplify this routine by making up several cotton balls at once and storing them in an air-tight jar.

Make sure that the essential oils are pure oil and plant (fruit, spice or flower). Chemically derived scents are potential allergens. Avoid adult scents like lavender which may contain estrogens or other elements not meant for children. You can find essential oils in health food stores. An online source is www.EssentialOil.com.

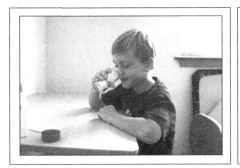 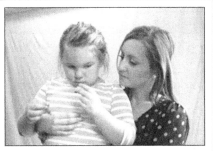 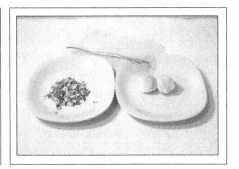

| **A boy sniffs essential oil on a cotton ball in a jar.** | **Girl smells a fresh herb.** | **Dried citrus or vanilla on cotton balls can also be used** |

Listening to music

The child listens to classical music once a day for 15 minutes using a portable CD player or music device and headphones (see the materials list, below).

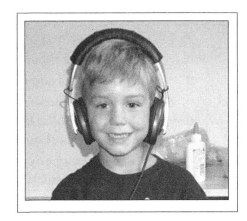

The original study used the album, *Classical Music for People Who Hate Classical Music, Vol. 1,* on the Direct Source label. In fact, there are many albums of classical music for children available online and in resale shops. Also consider other types of soft instrumental music, ethnic or folk instrumental music, and ambient music. Avoid music with a strong bass line which can be harmful to a child's ears. When possible, rotate through several different albums and set the music player to play the cuts randomly so that the child does not tire of or obsess on individual pieces.

Selecting and obtaining music and headphones

CDs are easily found in resale shops, your local library and online. If you can manage it, get several albums, avoiding overlapping content.

We want the child to listen to the music over headphones. The quality of his listening experience will be affected by the quality of the headphones. Look for headphones that fit well and that have a mellow sound. You may find good used headphones in a resale shop or online.

To introduce headphones to the child, plug them into the TV and then put on the child's favorite cartoons. Explain that the sound is now in the headphones. Most children will put on the headphones to hear their cartoon, and in the process, adapt to the headphones. Optionally, the child can listen over speakers.

Materials for the Activities

Materials needed for the exercises are listed below. For the most part, they are easily found at home, in school and in resale shops. You don't need all of the items at once, so focus on locating materials you will need within the next month. You will want to look through the alternate exercises ("easier activities" and "harder activities") to see what additional items might be useful.

Many of the items are bulky. Try to keep your materials organized in bags and bins so that the program doesn't fall apart due to loss of key items.

Here are the materials needed for all 34 activities. **Note that the short version exercises are indicated in bold.**

Activities	Materials
1	**Three or four bowls, buckets or bins large enough to fit hands or feet; water of different temperatures.**
2	**Objects of different shapes and textures (hard, soft, smooth, rough, or fuzzy) for the child to touch and squeeze.**
3	**None.**
4	**Scarf or blindfold; materials of different textures to use as a walking pathway such as carpet, tile, wood, bubble wrap, and plastic mat.**
5	**Calm or classical music, music player, headphones or speakers.**
6	**Pillowcase; doubles of small common objects like keys, coins, unsharpened pencils, small toys, stones, pine cones, spoons, and so on.**
7	Naturally scented bath salts, soaps and oils; bathtub. Alternatively: scented lotion.
8	Two spoons; a cup of very hot water and a cup of very cold water.
9	**Two spoons; a cup of very hot water and a cup of very cold water.**
10	**Objects and pictures of the objects. For small children use actual images such as printed photos or photos taken and displayed on a phone or tablet. For older children, drawings of the objects should work.**
11	**Blindfold; a wooden plank for walking on such as a board that is approximately two inches (5 cm) thick, eight inches (20 cm) wide and about five feet (1.5 m) long.**
12	**Ice cubes, large colorful beads; bowl or plate.**
13	**A book with pictures; bell, buzzer or other sound maker.**
14	**Several bowls filled with water of different temperatures; a few small objects to put in the bowls.**
15	**Buttons large and small.**
16	Large pillows, foam or a sleeping bag.
17	**Books with pictures of objects the child is familiar with.**
18	A cool and a warm object. (Cups of water will work.)
19	Grains of rice, dough (see dough recipes in the sensory chapter, touch-desensitization section).

Activities	Materials
20	Small 2x2 inch (5x5 cm) squares of differently textured materials: plastic, cardboard, carpet, bubble wrap, aluminum foil, etc.
21	Textured objects as in exercises 2 and 20.
22	Ice-filled straws or ice cubes, double wrapped in plastic wraps.
23	A tray or plate that has been chilled. Use metal or non-breakable glass if available.
24	None.
25	Piggy bank, coins, large cardboard box or three-fold display board (like those used for science projects). You will need to construct a viewing device. The instructions can be found in Enrichment 25.
26	Purchased or home-made magnetic pole; paper clips.
27	Letter-paper sized picture; red object such as a red-marker cap or very large bead.
28	Stairs; pillow or bolster.
29	Paper and pencil.
30	Two pencils; paper.
31	**Pictures or a book of colorful pictures; colored beads.**
32	Small feather; small pieces of aluminum foil.
33	Two or more postcard-sized pictures.
34	Music from other countries or music with a theme; books showing pictures of the theme.

CHAPTER 4

Enrichment Exercises
and Related Activities

This chapter contains the original 34 exercises (long version) of the Environmental Enrichment protocol plus supplemental graded activities for children of different abilities. Individual activities can be performed as part of the Environmental Enrichment protocol or used separately as an intervention for a child with specific sensory problems.

Therapy goals for performing each activity are listed at the start of each exercise and can be used by therapists, teachers and parents to select activities. Each exercise lists the materials needed, precise instructions for doing the exercise, safety considerations, sensory considerations, as well as easier and harder alternate exercises.

Read the instructions found in chapter 3 before beginning the protocol.

Hands in Water

Activity: Place hands and feet in water of different temperatures

Goals: To increase thermal awareness; to integrate thermal and touch sensation processing.

Materials: Four bowls, pails or basins containing water of different temperatures: hot, warm, cool, cold. The bowls can be labeled *hot, warm, cool* and *cold*. Consider color coding the labels or the bowls: hot is red, warm is pink, cool is light blue, and cold is bright blue.

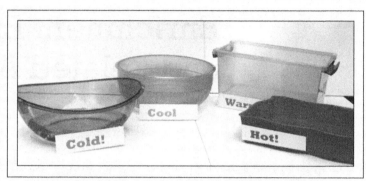

Put water in four bowls that are large enough to fit a hand or foot; label bowls and play!

Instructions: Have the child put his hands or feet into the bowls to feel water of different temperatures. Encourage the child to play and splash in the water. Say the words, *hot, warm, cool* or *cold* as the child feels the water. Play simple games. For example, place his hands in cold water and playfully ask, "Is it hot?", and encourage the answer, "NO! It's cold!"

For starters, put just a small amount of water in each bowl, and then gradually increase the amount over the two-week period.

Safety considerations: Avoid water temperatures that are too hot or cold.

Sensory considerations: If the child does not like the sensation of water, try using sand, uncooked rice, or beans instead. Heat or cool them to the appropriate temperatures. (See activities and cautions in the "easier activities" below.)

To reduce sensitivity, try massaging fingers or toes prior to having him put them in water. (Read the desensitization section of chapter 1, and the section on touch desensitization in chapter 6.) For serious concerns, consult an occupational therapist.

Easier Activities:

- Place finger into a small puddle of water on the table. Encourage the child to rub his hand or foot in it.
- On the first day, fill just one bowl with water the temperature of bathwater. Gradually add bowls of water of different temperatures, increasing the temperatures of the warm bowls and decreasing the temperatures of the cool bowls over time.
- Dip finger into a small cup of warm water, then into a small cup of cool water. Do this until the child is willing to do it herself. Gradually increase the size of the bowl and the temperatures.

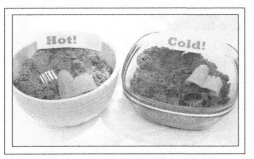

Sand is a good alternative for a child who is fearful of water.

- **Play in warm sand and cool sand, rice, or beans.** To do this, put sand (rice or beans) in glass or ceramic bowls. Put one bowl in the refrigerator to cool. Heat another (oven-proof) bowl in a warm oven until very warm but not too hot. A few minutes prior to the exercise, put another bowl in the oven so that it is slightly warm. The fourth bowl can be at room temperature. Set out labels for the dishes (*hot, warm, cool, cold*). Have the child play in the bowls with feet or hands.

<u>Caution:</u> If you use sand, take care that it is from a known source or is graded as "children's play sand." Cover and store the bowls and sand for future use.

Harder Activities:

- Play outside, bringing the child's awareness to the temperature of things in the environment.
- **Snow balls:** On a snowy day, make snowballs, catch falling snow on tongues, drink hot chocolate, have the child put a hand on your neck to feel the warmth.
- **Mud puddles (or garden hoses):** On a hot day make a puddle (or fill a plastic bin) with a garden hose. Feel hot concrete, put bare feet in a puddle or bin, drink ice water.

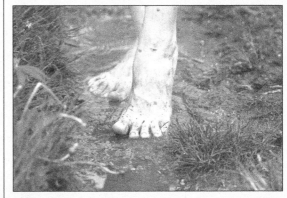

A cool mud puddle on a warm day is a perfect way to feel hot and cold at the same time.

- **Stack hot and cold pennies. (See photo.)** Set out two small bowls containing water—one with ice water, the other with hot, (but comfortable to the touch) water. Divide 30-40 pennies between the two bowls. (For children with poor fine motor skills, use larger coins like nickels or quarters.) Play one of the games listed below:

  o Have the child stack pennies, alternating hot or cold pennies. Encourage the child to continue stacking until at last the stack tumbles.

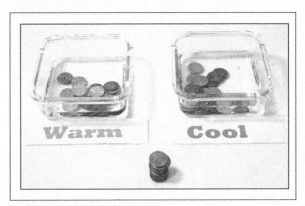

Coins are place in hot and cold water for the child to retrieve and place in a tall stack.

  o To further increase the challenge, have the child simultaneously get a hot and cold coin using two hands. Stack them.

  o Switch bowl positions each time so that the child's hands are alternately immersed in hot and cold water.

  o Use a mixture of coins (pennies, nickels, dimes, and quarters) for a greater challenge in stacking

<u>Caution:</u> Small objects hazard.

- **Make a racket with homemade drums and cymbals, and hot and cold spoons.** Gather a variety of makeshift "drums and cymbals": lids, jars (some partially filled with water), cans and an oatmeal box. Use hot and cold spoons as drum sticks. Now, make a racket! Replace the spoons with fresh ones when they lose their temperature. To dampen the noise, put pots and lids on towels. Use a simple social story like the one below to create a context for this type of play.

  Story: "I'm happy! Let's play "make a racket"! Here is a warm spoon, beat on the lid with the spoon. Now quick, get a cold spoon, beat on the pot with that. Yea! It's fun to make a racket! Now let's be quiet. Can you tap softly? . . ."

- **Make a drawing with ice cold veggies and heated grains.** Heat grains of rice, beans and lentils until they are very warm, place them in a dish labeled "hot." Place small amounts of colorful frozen vegetable and berries into a bowl labeled "cold." Lay out paper towels to draw on, and invite the child to draw a person, animal, house or car using the hot and cold materials. Coach him in making the picture by asking leading questions: "How many arms does he have?" "What color is the roof?" "Does your dog have ears? Where do they go?" Start the picture for him if he does not initiate himself.

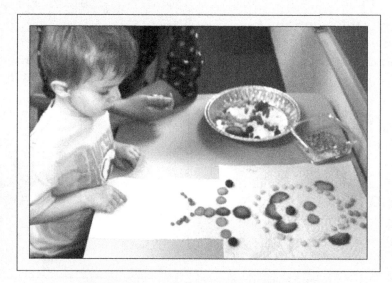

Child draws a boy using frozen peas, corn, berries and warm beans and rice.

Play with Textures

Activity: Squeeze objects of different shapes and textures

Goals: To integrate touch, vision and motor; to increase fine motor skills.

Materials: Squeezable items, toys, food, and household items with different textures. Include hard items such as wood, stone and plastic; soft items such as fleece and yarn; mushy foods like bananas and berries; and squishy items such as a rubber duck or a Nerf™ ball.

Activities: Create simple games that allow the child to explore textures. Name the sensations and textures: soft, mushy, hard, cold, juicy, watery, silky or icky. Ask if she likes the way it feels.

- Wrap yarn or soft wire around a spool or small round container.
- Line up stones or marbles.
- Fill a squirt gun or rubber duck with water and squeeze.
- Squeeze fruits. (Have a bowl of rinsing water nearby so that the child can explore gooey textures and then clean up.)
- Wrap string around hand, arm or finger.
- In the kitchen, investigate foods and make a game of finding different textures – sponge, cloth, pan or spoon, plastic, vegetables.
- Stack wood blocks or logs.
- Investigate indoor or outdoor plants.

Safety considerations: Monitor the child when using yarn, string, wire and ribbon. Avoid a choking hazard by using large objects if the child puts things into her mouth.

Sensory considerations: If the child is unable to handle the texture of squeezing fruit, play a game in which she touches it quickly and then wipes it off her finger. See the desensitization section of chapter 1, and the section on touch desensitization in chapter 6.

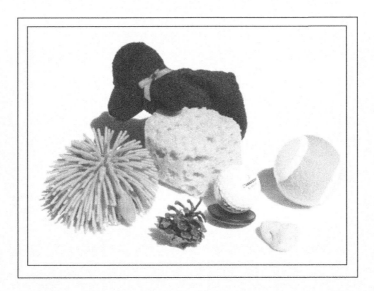

Easier Activities:

- Press textured objects into the child's hand and wrap her fingers around them. Say, "This is a [object name] it feels [soft, hard, mushy . . .]."
- Put an object on the table, with your hand over the child's hand, help her pick it up, saying, "Pick up the [object name]."
- Put the object onto the table and tell her to pick it up. Once the object is in her hand, tell her to squeeze it.

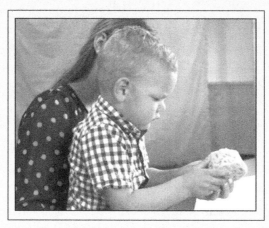

Harder Activities:

- There are many ways to investigate and enjoy textures including these:
  o Make a yarn doll
  o Make balls and snakes with dough
  o Shoot marbles
  o Make mountains in sandboxes

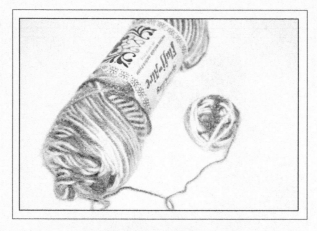

The texture of yarn is soothing. Have the child engage in activities such as rolling balls of yarn and making yarn dolls.

Sensation on Face and Arms

Activity: Draw imaginary lines on the child's face and arms

Goals: To increase touch awareness; to desensitize to light touch; to register touch; to integrate touch and vision.

Materials: None needed.

Instructions: Tell the child that you are going to touch his arm with your finger. Draw lines on the child's face, legs and arms. Vary the pressure of the touch. Start with a firm touch and eventually move to a feather-light touch. Talk about what you are drawing and how much pressure you are using. Later, ask him, "Is this a hard touch or a soft touch?" "How many lines did I draw?" "Is this a line or a circle?"

Safety considerations: Be aware that light touch can cause a defensive reaction in some children and cause them to react physically.

Sensory considerations: If the child is tactile defensive (acts with behaviors when touched), then consider first doing some strenuous play or aerobic exercise. Or have him hold and carry a heavy object like a weighted ball for about a minute. Use 1-2 pounds (.5-1 kilogram) weight for a toddler, up to 5 pounds (2 kilograms) for an 8-year-old and up to 10-12 pounds (4-6 kilograms) for older children.

In addition, try the easier activities listed below and make a note to share this information with the child's team. Many sensory therapists are knowledgeable about therapeutic interventions for children with tactile defensiveness.

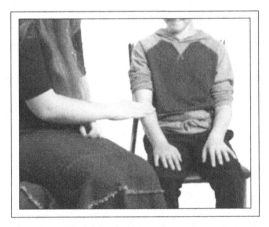

**Adult firmly touches
the child's arm**

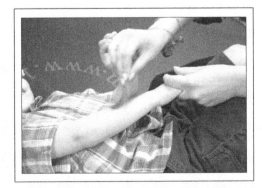

**Adult draws a line on the child's arm with a feather.
Use the nib of the feather for a firm line. Use the feather
hairs to give a light touch—as an advanced exercise.**

Easier Activities:

- Massage the skin firmly prior to drawing on it.
- Lay your hand flat on the child's arm firmly (or hold his arm firmly in your hand) for a few seconds then move your hand up and down on the arm, pressing firmly. Repeat on the other arm, and then on different areas of the face. This will help to decrease the irritation from the touch of materials.
- Here are ways to acclimate the child to touch, try these in the order given:

  o Press your finger firmly on the child's arm and leave it there for a few seconds.

  o Press your finger on the skin and draw a short line with firm pressure.

  o Use your finger to firmly draw lines on the child's skin.

  o Repeat the above steps on the face and legs.

Harder Activities:

- Draw lines with a lighter touch. If the child is defensive, rub out the spot you touched. Show him how to rub it out, too.
- Draw lines with a feather touch.
- Move to the activities in Enrichment 5.

Walk on Textures Blindfolded

Activity: Walk on a pathway of different textures blindfolded

Goals: To increase vestibular (balance) skills; to increase the sense-of-touch touch registration of novel materials; to integrate the touch and vestibular senses.

Materials: A scarf or sash for a blindfold; a walkway of textured surfaces. When working indoors include some combination of carpet, tile, wood, area rugs, shag carpet, fiber mats, rubber mats (see note), plastic mats, fake grass, thin bubble wrap and other textured materials. Lay them in a row on the floor near a wall that can be used for support. When working outdoors, incorporate grass, dirt, mud puddles and paved surfaces into the textured path.

Instructions: Create a path of textured materials near a wall. Place a blindfold on the child and have her walk on surfaces with different textures in bare feet. Have her use the wall for balance. If walking blindfolded proves to be too difficult, have her walk first without the blindfold. Once she is accustomed to this exercise, name the textures a second or two after she has stepped on them. Consider labeling each material: "wool, wood, tile, plastic," and reciting the label names with her before and after the exercise.

Safety considerations: Ensure that mats are secure to the floor and do not pose a trip hazard to the child. **Do Not Use Rubber Materials If The Child Has a Latex Allergy.** Some children lose balance when they are blindfolded and so should try just a step or two at a time.

Sensory considerations: If wearing a blindfold is too difficult, ask her to close her eyes or cover her eyes with your hand. The easier exercises listed below should be helpful for children who do not tolerate bare feet. Children who crave bare feet will enjoy the harder exercises. However, if a child prefers bare feet because she does not tolerate the sensation of socks and shoes, you will need to eventually work on touch desensitization. This is covered in my previous book, *Self-Regulation Interventions and Strategies*.

Easier Activities:

- Keep shoes on to walk across the novel path, then walk the path in stocking feet.
- Try rubbing feet or pressing firmly on the sole and arches to decrease the irritation from light touch of materials like carpet.
- Take one step onto a new surface and stand there.
- Try to get the child to accidently step on the mat by standing on it yourself while holding a favorite object of hers. Ask her to come and get it. Don't draw attention to the mat.
- Spread the mats around and make a game of jumping or hopping onto the surfaces.
- If the child appears fearful of a surface, place a favorite toy on it and let her retrieve it in her own time.

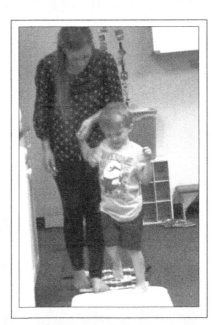

A boy is gingerly walking a textured pathway and holding the hand of an adult for balance.

- Try just one novel surface at a time and try easier ones first such as:
  - o Indoor-outdoor carpet
  - o Newspaper
  - o Bath mat, bath rug
  - o Plush carpet
  - o Vinyl, wood flooring
  - o Sand, soft dirt
  - o Playground mixture
- Try two or three surfaces at a time.
- Try each of the above in stocking feet then in bare feet.

Harder Activities:

- Try each of these in bare feet:
  - o Cold tile, slate, marble
  - o Grass
  - o Cement (for a short distance)
  - o Polished stone porch or walkway
  - o Rough welcome mat
  - o Brick walk
- Increase the distance, for example, walk across a yard or play in a park with bare feet.

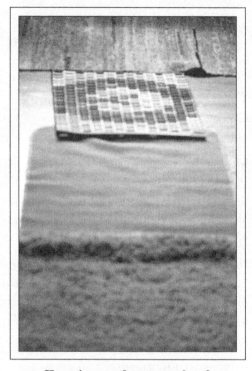

Here is a pathway made of a braided rug, a rough woven mat, a bathmat turned to the latex backing side, and a plush rug.

Sensation on Face and Arms with Music

Activity: Draw lines on the child's face, arms, and legs with objects while listening to music

Goals: To increase touch awareness; to desensitize to light touch; to register touch; to integrate touch and vision; to integrate touch and hearing.

Materials: None

Instructions: Play quiet music in the background. Tell the child that you are going to touch his arm with your finger. Next, firmly draw a line on the child's arm. Avoid soft touch until the child is comfortable with the exercise. Draw other lines on his arms, face and legs. Before you draw a line, tell him where you are going to draw it. Over time, make the touch lighter until it is a soft touch.

Safety considerations: None.

Sensory considerations: See Exercise 3. If a child is ticklish, put pressure on an area of the skin before drawing on it. Tell the child he can "rub it out" when you are done. A note on tickling: Honor the child who requests that you stop, while acknowledging his reaction, "Did that tickle? I'll draw harder so that it doesn't tickle you."

Loud and unexpected noises and soft or unexpected touch can trigger the fight-flight system, and cause the child to respond with defensive (and possibly aggressive) behaviors. Listening therapy programs are available for purchase, which have shown to help reduce this reaction. In addition, Therapressure™, a "brushing" technique with level-2 evidence, has been shown to help some children. Informal exercises, like this enrichment, in which sound and touch are integrated, can help the child acclimate to sound and touch. Try both the easier and harder activities listed below, as well.

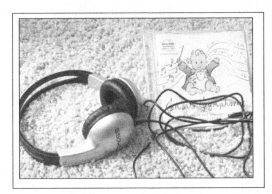
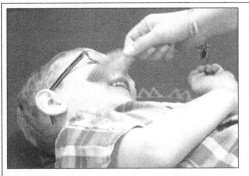

Easier Activities:

- See Enrichment 3 for easier touch activities.
- Play music softly in the background over speakers for a minute or two prior to introducing the drawing activity.

Harder Activities:

- See Enrichment 3 for harder touch activities.
- Try listening to music over headphones. (See the section titled *Listening to music* in the introduction to environmental enrichment.)
- Vary the type of music, avoiding music with a strong bass. (Or turn off the bass on the music device.)
- Attempt to draw lines on skin with soft objects. Stop if the child shows discomfort.
- Attempt to draw lines on skin with a light touch of the fingers. Stop if the child shows discomfort.
- If the child startles easily, talk about keeping his "ears turned on" so that he hears the warning signs of someone approaching. Use a story or the poem below to help make the point.
- Play with other children controlling bumping and noise until the child gets used to these factors. Gradually increase the intensity of play so that the child is exposed to the normal "rough and tumble" play of children.

Here's a poem that can be recited in a singsong voice to help the child become more alert to auditory cues.

I Keep My Ears Open

I love to watch my cartoon shows
I love to play with my Legos
But when I do, I'm telling you
I keep my ears open! I keep my ears open!

When my ears are shut tight, sounds give me a fright
I don't know who's where, and suddenly I scare
When my ears are open wide, people sounds get inside
I hear you coming; I know you're there

I love to watch my cartoon shows
I love to play with my Legos
But when I do, I'm telling you
I keep my ears open! I keep my ears open!

Enrichment 6
Match Object in Pillowcase

Activity: Find the twin of an object in a pillowcase

Goals: To help the child to recognize objects by touch only (increase stereognosis skills); integration of visual processing and touch processing.

Materials: A set of duplicate items small enough to put into a pillowcase such as keys, unsharpened pencils, spoons, buttons and small toys; labels for each object. Use items with different shapes, sizes and textures; optionally, an open bin filled with pom-pom balls to hide small objects in.

Instructions: Place one each of the duplicate objects into a pillow case. Show a twin object to the child and ask him to locate it in the pillowcase without looking. Display the object's name on a small card as it is shown to the child to help with language comprehension skills. Ask the child to repeat the name of the object.

Safety considerations: Avoid using sharp objects.

Sensory considerations: Only gradually introduce objects or materials that the child finds noxious. For a child with low vision, place objects in an open bin containing filler such as small pom-pom balls. This is a good exercise for helping the child to recognize items in the environment.

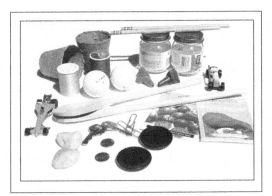

Use a wide variety of objects so that the child learns to identify different textures and shapes by touch.

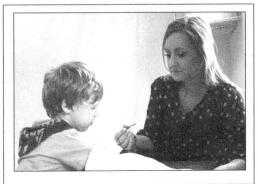

A boy tries to find a key among objects in a pillowcase.

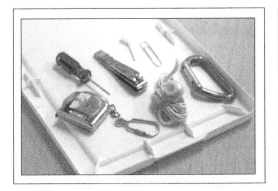

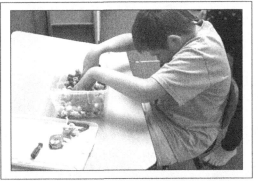

For a child with low vision, hide everyday objects in bins of beads, pom-pom balls, popcorn, beans, torn rags, coins or shredded paper. This will help him learn to recognize items by touch in his natural environment.

Easier Activities:

- Explore the characteristics of items one by one. Is it warm or cold to the touch; hard or soft; bumpy or smooth; big or small?
- Put one object in a pillowcase and place its twin plus several other objects on the table. Ask the child to identify the item in the pillowcase.
- Repeat the previous exercise, but with 2-3 items in the pillowcase. Slowly increase the number of items in the bag.

Harder Activities:

- Use pairs of items that are slightly different such as two cars of different sizes or two different types of markers.
- Put the items into a bin filled with pom-pom balls or beans—as described in the materials section above. Name an item for the child to locate.

Scented Bath and Massage

Activity: Take a scented bath and a get a massage with scented oil or scented lotion

Once the child adapts to this exercise, it can be used as part of a bedtime calming routine.

Goals: To provide the soothing input of combined scent and touch; to integrate smell and touch.

Materials: Naturally scented bath salts, soaps and oils. Use child-friendly scents like fruits or flowers. You can make a batch of scented oil by putting a drop or two of essential oil into a small bottle of jojoba oil. Optionally, purchase natural scented oils and soaps, or purchase jojoba oil and bath salts, in health food stores and online.

For the alternate exercise, use a lightly scented lotion. If the lotion you have is too strongly scented, mix it with an unscented lotion to the desired intensity.

Alternate exercise: If the program is being done in a school environment, apply (or for older children, have the child apply) lightly scented lotion.

Instructions: Add a drop or two of essential oil to the child's bath. Following the bath, give the child a massage with scented oil.

Safety considerations: Use only natural scents. To check for allergic reactions, put a dab of new oils or diluted salts on a small area of the child's arm 24 hours prior to using it in the bath. Look for rashes, fevers or other indications of allergic reaction.

Sensory considerations: Ask the child which scents he prefers.

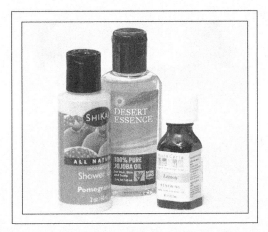

There are many natural options for bath scents.
Consider making your own bath oil using grapeseed oil, sweet almond oil
or jojoba oil with a few drops of the child's favorite scent.

Bonus Activity: Make Bath Bombs

Bath bombs are a fun way to enjoy a fragrant bath. Hide a small toy in the bomb and see the surprise on the child's face when it appears in the fizzing water! Hot water (not cold water) activates the bombs. A small child can help in making the bombs if you first wrap sandwich bags around his hands before he "mushes" the mixture and forms the bombs.

Ingredients:

1 1/2 cup baking soda

1/2 cup citric acid powder (available online and where canning supplies are sold)

Grapeseed oil or Sweet almond oil

Essential oil(s) for scent

Small toys

Optional: food coloring

Optional: craft molds (available at craft stores)

Mix the dry ingredients.

(You can make a large batch of the dry ingredients and store what you don't use in a tight container.)

1. Put a sieve over a bowl. Put the baking soda and citric acid through the sieve.
2. Mix well with a whisk.

Make the bombs:

1. In a small bowl, add ½ tsp. of grapeseed oil or sweet almond oil, 4-6 drops of essential oil and (if you are using it) about 10 drops of food coloring.
2. Add ½ cup of the baking soda and citric acid mixture and mix well using your fingers to ensure that it is mixed well. (Use gloves if you are using food coloring.)
3. Place a small toy in the center of the mixture and firmly press the mixture in the bowl flat. Optionally, place the toy and mixture into a craft mold.
4. Gently slip the bomb out of the bowl and upside down onto a flat container. It will be dome shaped. If you are using a mold, remove the bomb from the mold.
5. Continue making bombs until your batch is used up. Store the bombs for 36 hours before using.

Attention to Sound and Temperature

Activity: While speaking or singing, touch arms and legs with a cooled or warmed spoon

Goals: To acclimate to being touched by objects in the environment; to decrease fight-flight reaction from random touch; to integrate touch and sound.

Materials: Two spoons and a source for heating and cooling the spoons such as cups containing hot and ice cold water.

Instructions: Pour hot water into one cup and cold water into another. Place spoons into them and let them sit for a minute or so. Check the spoon's temperature then place one spoon on the child's leg or arm while talking or singing to the child. Put that spoon back into its cup and switch spoons. Continue doing this for several minutes.

Safety considerations: Take care with the water temperature. As mentioned, be aware that light touch can cause a defensive reaction in some children and cause them to physically react.

Sensory considerations: If the child has tactile defensiveness, start each session by pressing the spoons firmly to the skin prior to lightening the touch. Also read the *sensory considerations* sections in Enrichments 3 and 5.

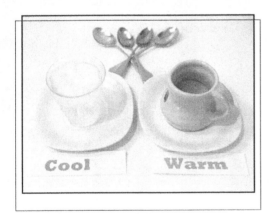

Ice water and hot water for chilling and warming the spoons.

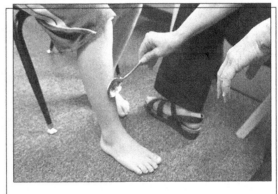

Adult placing spoon on child's leg while speaking to the child.

Easier Activities:

- See the easier activities for Enrichment 5 for sound and touch.

Harder Activities:

- See the harder activities for Enrichment 5 for sound and touch.
- In a group setting, sit in a circle and pass a cool object, then a warm object from child to child. Repeat this with a warm sandbag, potato or stone.
- Play toss with a chilled orange or apple. For younger children, roll an orange or apple on the floor back and forth.

Body Sensation and Temperature

Activity: Draw lines on arms and legs with cooled or warmed spoons

Goals: To help the child to acclimate to temperature and to objects touching her; to help with touch discrimination as the line is drawn.

Materials: Two spoons and a source for heating and cooling the spoons such as cups containing very hot and very cold water.

Instructions: Pour hot water into a cup and place a spoon into it. Pour ice water into another cup and put the other spoon into it. Let them sit for a minute or so. Check the spoon's temperature, then when the temperature is right, draw lines on the child's skin. As in Enrichment 5, vary the pressure of the touch. Start with a firm touch and eventually move to a feather-light touch. Put the spoon back into its cup and switch spoons. Continue doing this for several minutes.

Safety considerations: Take care with the hot water and keep it out of a young child's reach. Again, remember that light touch can create a defensive reaction in some children and cause them to physically react.

Sensory considerations: If the child has tactile defensiveness, be sure to press the spoons firmly onto the skin.

Easier Activities:

- See Enrichments 1 and 8 for easier hot and cold activities.
- See Enrichment 3 for easier touch activities.

Harder Activities:

- See Enrichments 1 and 8 for harder hot and cold activities.
- See Enrichments 3 and 5 for harder touch activities.
- For overall temperature tolerance, have the child help with functional activities such as:
  - o Passing small warm or cool bowls of food at the dinner table
  - o Carrying wet towels from the bathroom
  - o Carrying clothes fresh from the dryer
  - o Helping to get fruit from a bin in the refrigerator
- Make a walking version of tag called "apple tag" in which children tag with a chilled object such as a small apple.

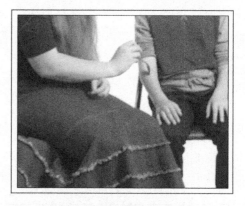

Adult drawing line on child's arm with a spoon.

Visual Matching Pictures & Objects

Activity: Match a picture of an object to the real object

Goals: To increase object identification skills, attention skills; visual discrimination; integrate vision and motor.

Materials: A collection of objects plus pictures of them. For example, if you are using a book with pictures of fruit, you will need a set of matching real or plastic fruit. Optionally, create a collection of objects and take photos of them. You may want to print the photos (as opposed to showing them on a phone or tablet) to decrease the chance of the child being distracted by electronics.

Instructions: Put a collection of objects near the child. Ask him to look at a picture of one of the objects and point to the actual object. If this task is too easy for him, consider finding objects that have a similar appearance so that he must match subtler features of the objects. Ask him to name the objects.

Safety considerations: Avoid very small objects with a child who is young or puts things in his mouth.

Sensory considerations: None.

Easier Activities:

- Use photos (which are easy for a concrete thinker) instead of images.
- Start with photos of yourself and of the child. Show a picture of him and ask him to point to who it is. Next show him a picture of you.
- Limit to two or three objects on the table for him to choose from.

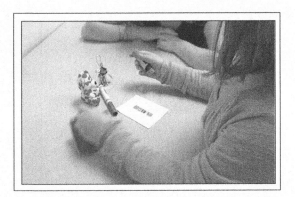

Harder Activities:

- Line up pictures of objects on a table, and then have the child place each object on top of its photo.
- Instead of using a picture, use oral commands. Say the name of one of the objects and ask the child to point to it.
- See Enrichment 17.

Walk a Plank

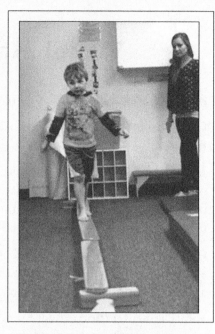

Activity: Walk on a 2 × 8-inch × 5-foot plank with eyes open, then blindfolded

A child's ability to balance while walking on a plank may change dramatically with a blindfold. Some children lose balance when they are blindfolded, while others can walk blindfolded but are unable to do as well without the blindfold. In either case, practice is typically all that is needed to increase skills.

Goals: To increase vestibular (balance) skills; to improve attention and focus skills; to integrate vision and vestibular senses.

Materials: A board approximately two inches (5 centimeters) thick, eight inches (20 centimeters) wide and about five feet (1.5 meters) long. A four-inch-wide (10 centimeter) board may work and will be a greater challenge for an older child. Boards longer than five feet can be used, but may be more difficult to store.

Instructions: Place a wooden plank on the floor near a wall for support. Ask the child to walk the length of the plank. Blindfold her, and then ask her to walk it again. (This exercise begs for stories of pirates walking the plank – but only after the child has achieved success. See poem at the end of this exercise.)

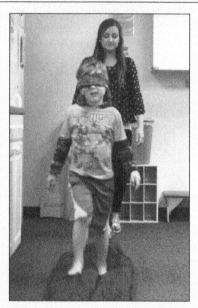

Safety considerations: The board should not be more than two inches thick so that children who are unsteady will not hurt themselves if they lose balance.

Sensory considerations: If this is too difficult for the child, start with walking between two lines on the floor. Make the lines closer and closer together until the child can manage a width of eight inches. Next, move to a one-inch thick board and finally to the two-inch board. (See the easier instructions.)

Easier Activities:

For some children, this activity may be quite difficult. In this section, the process has been broken down into small, easier steps.

- Walk a line:
  o Place a circle or 'x' on the floor (near a wall) with masking tape or string and ask the child to stand on it. A circle will be conceptually easier for the child.
  o Draw a line on the floor, six-feet long. Place an 'x' or a circle at each end. Ask the child to walk on the line from one 'x' to the other. Hold her hand and steady her, if necessary.

- To increase acceptance of the blindfold:
    - o Put a blindfold over your eyes and laugh. Then tell the child it's her turn.
    - o Use a treat or social reward such as a hug to help her accept the blindfold.
    - o Place your hand over her eyes.
    - o Use a paper bag instead of a blindfold.
- Walk the line blindfolded:
    - o Demonstrate walking the line with the blindfold over your eyes. Ask the child to hold your hand as you do it.
    - o Place the blindfold on the child and hold her hand as she walks on the line.
- Getting used to the board and the blindfold:
    - o Place the board on the floor near a wall. Have the child stand on the board.
    - o Have the child walk the length of the board.
    - o Have the child stand on the board blindfolded.
    - o Hold the child's hand, and then have her walk the length of the board with the blindfolded.

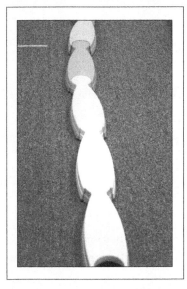

Two inch (5cm) high blocks that can be assembled for a walking path

Harder Activities:

- Carry an object while walking a line. A long object such as a yardstick (or meterstick) will help with balance.
- Carry a smaller object while walking the board.
- Carry a smaller object while walking the board blindfolded.
- Enrichment 16.

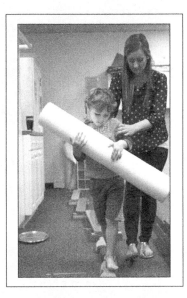

Child carrying a large object while walking on a board

I WALK THE PLANK

My eyes, they are blind
Still I walk a straight line,
With body straight and tall
And steps very small

My arms are stretched wide
And sway side-to-side
And so I don't fall,
I can touch the wall

I walk the plank true
I walk it fast, too
No pirate at sea
Walks it better than me

Pick Beads from Ice

Activity: Remove a colored bead from a dish filled with ice cubes

Goals: To improve visual discrimination, fine motor skills, and touch or thermal sensory integration.

Materials: 8-12 ice cubes; one or more colored beads; a flat dish. Grade the skill level needed for this exercise by increasing or decreasing the size of the beads.

Instructions: Put ice and one colorful bead on a flat dish. Have the child pick the bead from the dish. When the child is successful at performing this exercise, consider placing several beads on the plate.

Safety considerations: If the child has poor temperature sensation, be sure that he does not hold onto ice cubes for more than a few seconds.

Sensory considerations: If you suspect the child is color blind, use a bright or dark colored bead.

Easier Activities:

- If the ice causes problems, use clear beads or tempered-glass stones in place of the ice.
- Pick a red bead out of a bowl of yellow or white beads.
- Put beads in a dish with a small amount of chilled water. Have the child pick them out of the dish.
- Enrichments 8, 9, 18.

Harder Activities:

- Enrichment 22.

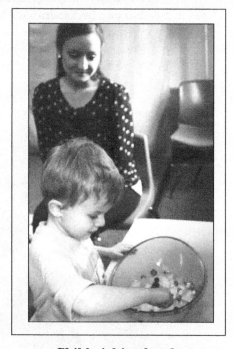

**Child picking beads
from a bowl of ice**

Attention to Sound

Activity: Use a sound cue to distract attention away from a visual task

Goals: To increase attention to sound cues and to speaking.

Materials: Photos or a book of pictures; a bell, buzzer or small gong.

Instructions: Show the child a picture, then ring a bell and say her name or a phrase such as, "look at me."

Safety considerations: None.

Sensory considerations: Choose a bell or sound that is not annoying to the child.

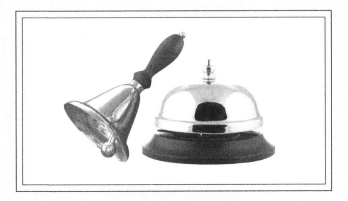

Bells for cueing

Easier Activities:

- While the child looks at the picture, ring the bell and gently touch her hand or her face while saying, "Look at me." Optionally use a reward to reinforce this.
- Create a small story such as the following and read it to the child: "I like to look at books. But I also need to pay attention to the sounds around me. When I hear a bell or hear [mom, my teacher, Miss Rita] call my name, I need to look at [mom, my teacher, Miss Rita] and see what she wants."
- Read the poem in Enrichment 5, "I Keep My Ears Open."

Harder Activities:

- Get the child's attention by saying her name without ringing the bell.
- Get the child's attention by ringing the bell without saying her name.
- If the child is annoyed by a bell or buzzer sound, record the sound and play it in the background at a reduced (and comfortable) volume several times a day. Slowly turn up the volume.

Enrichment 14
Find Objects in Water

Activity: Remove objects from cool and warm bowls of water

Goals: To increase fine motor skills; improve thermal and touch integration.

Materials: Two bowls; small objects such as marbles, keys, or coins.

Instructions: Fill one bowl with warm (not hot) water, the other with cool water. Place small objects in each bowl. Have the child pick objects from bowls in succession. Replace the objects and repeat for several minutes.

Safety considerations: Ensure that water temperature is not too hot or cold. Small objects are a choking hazard.

Sensory considerations: None.

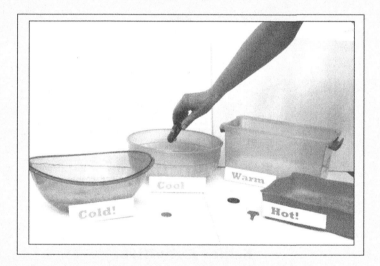

Put various objects in different water temperatures and have the child retrieve them.

Easier Activities:

- Enrichment 1.
- Use larger, easier-to-grasp objects.

Harder Activities:

- See the harder activities in Enrichment 1.
- Put small grains of rice or beans in the water.

Game: Find the coin

Materials: Cups, dish soap, coins

Instructions: Put water of different temperatures into small bowls. Add enough dish soap to make thick bubbles. Have the child swish the water to make bubbles in each bowl, and then hide a coin or "prize" in one of the bowls. Have the child look for the coin in each bowl.

Pull a Button from Fingers

Activity: Pull a button from between someone's fingers

Goals: To increase fine motor skills; to increase sensation of finger pressure.

Materials: Buttons of different sizes and colors.

Instructions: Start with a large, bright or dark colored button. Hold the button between your fingers. Tell the child to take it from you. Repeat this exercise using smaller and smaller buttons. Also, gradually use buttons of a lighter color. Once she is familiar with this procedure, have her put the button into a piggy bank or slotted jar.

Safety considerations: There is a small object hazard for children who put things in their mouths.

Sensory considerations: None.

Easier Activities:

- Pick up small objects.
- Enrichment 12: pick bead out of ice.
- Enrichment 14: remove objects from water.

Harder Activities:

- Button a large button.
- Zip a jacket.
- Button a small button through a loose hole.
- Button a small button through a tighter hole.
- Enrichment 25: put coins in a piggy bank using only a mirrored reflection of hands.

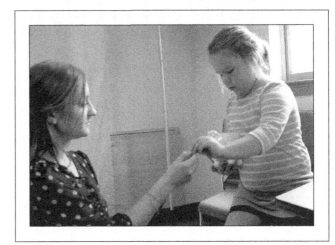

Pulling a button from an adult's hand.

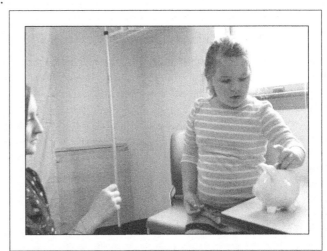

Girl takes a coin from the therapist and puts it into a piggy bank.

Walk on Bouncy Surface

Activity: Walk on a bouncy surface of foam or large pillows with eyes open, then blindfolded

Goals: To increase the ability to balance; improve attention-to-task.

Materials: Enough thick foam or pillows to make a three-to-five foot-long (1-1.5 meter) path. The foam should be about as thick as a pillow.

Instructions: Place foam, large pillows or a doubled-over sleeping bag on the floor near a wall for support. Have the child walk on them. When he can do this successfully, blindfold him and ask him to walk on them again.

Safety considerations: The foam or pillows should be challenging but feasible to walk on. Make sure the child moves slowly as he walks. Some children lose balance when they are blindfolded, and so they should try just a step or two at a time.

Sensory considerations: See Enrichment 11 for a discussion and strategies for balance (vestibular) issues.

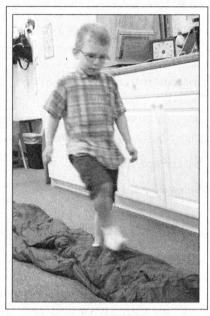

Boy walks along a rolled-up sleeping bag.

Easier Activities:

- Enrichments 4, 11.

Harder Activities:

- Walk across piles of blankets and towels.
- Walk across a large pillow made of large chunks of foam.
- Walk across an air mattress placed near a wall. Use wall for support.

Name Objects in Pictures

Activity: Point to objects in a picture and name them

Goals: To integrate motor and speech; increase cognition.

Materials: Books with pictures of objects.

Instructions: Have the child look at a page of pictures of objects. Then ask him to point out and name objects that he sees.

Safety considerations: None.

Sensory considerations: None.

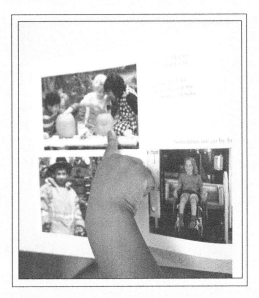

Girl points to a pumpkin in a picture.

Easier Activities:

- Enrichment 10: Match an object to its picture.
- Point to familiar objects on verbal command.

Harder Activities:

- Point to a line drawing of an object in a picture.
- Describe color, size or other features of the object.

More Attention to Temperature

Activity: Place a finger on a cool object, and then on a warm one

Goals: To increase thermal awareness and thermal discrimination; touch and thermal integration. This exercise can also be used as part of a safety lesson (with a story or video) for hot and cold.

Materials: Warm and cool objects. At home, these could consist of food fresh from the refrigerator or the microwave. In hot or cold weather heat or air vents and cold or warm windows work. For older children, the refrigerator itself or a warm stove suffice.

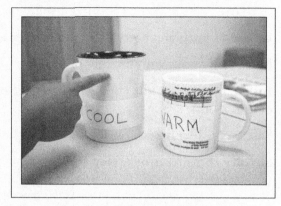

Touch a cool object then a warm one!

Instructions: Place the child's fingers on a cool object, and then on a warm object. Say the words "warm" and "cool" as the child's finger moves.

Safety considerations: Check an object's temperatures prior to having the child touch its surface.

Sensory considerations: Some children with autism process both pain and temperature slowly. The child may feel the heat or cold sensation only after several seconds have elapsed. Use objects that are hot and cold—but not so hot as to be unsafe—as they will register more easily. Exercises such as these can help to increase awareness and to decrease processing time.

Easier Activities:

- See Enrichments 8 and 9.

Harder Activities:

- At home, ask the child to help in the kitchen and touch cold, cool, warm and almost hot ingredients and foods.
- Write a story together or have a conversation about how cold things get warmer and hot things become cooler.

I Can Feel So Much!

Is it cold? Is it hot?
Is it warm? Is it not?
Is it cool to my touch?
I can feel so much!
When it's hot or very cold,
Stay away, I am told
Like the oven and the fire
And the freezer and the dryer
Like the pot and the pan
Or the backside of the fan
They can hurt me! I should learn
What is safe and what will burn
What is cold? What is hot?
What is safe? What is not?
Is it cool to my touch?
I can feel so very much!

Enrichment 19

Pick Up Rice

Activity: Create a small depression in dough and put rice into it

Goals: To increase fine motor skills and visual motor skills; integration of touch, vision and motor.

Materials: Dough or Play-Doh™; grains of rice, or small beans, peas or lentils. Recipes for dough are provided in the touch desensitization section of Chapter 6.

Instructions: Place a chunk of dough on a table. Have the child press a hole in it and then place grains of rice into the hole. If rice grains are too small for the child to manipulate, try using small beans, peas or lentils instead.

Safety considerations: Use edible dough if the child mouths objects.

Sensory considerations: If the texture of the dough is too gooey for the child, then put the rice grains into a bottle cap instead.

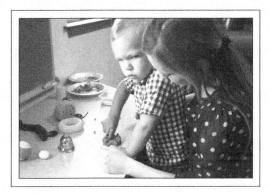

Roll the dough into a ball, then press the center to make a bowl.

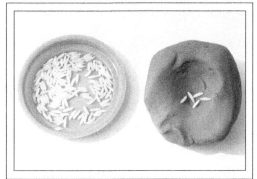

Place grains of rice into the bowl.

Easier Activities:

- Play with dough.
- Press dough into shapes.

Harder Activities:

- Create dough people or animals with rice and beans for eyes, mouth and nose.
- Create dough people or animals and make eyes, ears, nose and mouth from small pieces of different colored dough.

More Visual Matching

Activity: Select a textured square that matches its photo

Goals: To increase visual discrimination skills; integration of touch and vision.

Materials: A collection of 2x2 inch (5x5 centimeter) squares of different textures; photos of the squares. Squares can be cut from plastic mats, carpet, cardboard, bubble wrap, foam, aluminum foil, fine sandpaper, felt and sponge.

Instructions: Place the textured squares on the table. Show the child a photo of one of the squares and have her pick out and pick up the matching square.

Safety considerations: Avoid rubber if the child has a latex allergy.

Sensory considerations: Be aware of textures that the child does not wish to touch. Gradually expose the child to that texture.

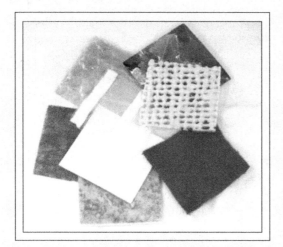 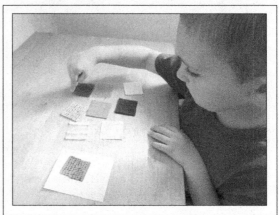

**Cut two-inch square tiles of differently textured materials.
Ask the child to match a photos of the tiles to the actual tiles.**

Easier Activities:

• Enrichment 2 and the harder activities listed there.

Harder Activities:

• Have the child say, write, type or point to a word that describes a texture such as fuzzy, scratchy, soft, hard, cool, and so on.
• Have the child name the color.
• Have the child identify what the texture is used for, such as, "That's carpet." Or "That's for curtains."

Enrichment 21

Sensation of Textures on Face

Activity: Draw imaginary circles on the child's face using textured objects

Goals: To increase sensory awareness of the skin; to increase cognitive awareness of textures.

Materials: Objects of different textures including small toys.

Instructions: Take turns using textured objects, including toys, foods and household items, to draw circles on the face of the child. Once he is comfortable with the process, ask him questions such as how big the circles are, whether they feel soft, hard or mushy, and what feels best.

Safety considerations: Keep an eye out for sharp surfaces on objects.

Sensory considerations: If the child displays defensiveness to touch, use a firm rather than a light stroke.

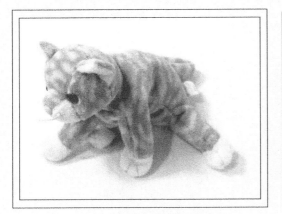 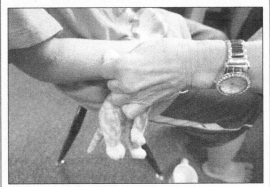

The paw of a small fuzzy toy animal works well for this exercise.

Easier Activities:

- Enrichments 3, 5.

Harder Activities:

- See the suggestions for harder activities in Enrichments 3 and 5.
- Ask the child to close his eyes and guess what you are using for drawing.

Play with Cold Objects

Activity: Places ice-filled straws into dough, alternating hands

Goals: To increase thermal sensory awareness; decrease thermal sensitivity; integrate touch, thermal and visual senses.

Materials: A chunk of dough or Play-Doh™; ice straws or straws filled with water and frozen. To fill straws with ice, cap one end with wax, dough or gum. Fill straw with water, and then set it upright in the freezer until the ice has frozen, or use a kitchen gadget called an ice straw maker to make ice straws. (It's found in kitchen shops and online). Optionally, freeze long green beans.

Instructions: Place a chunk of dough on the table. Have the child press ice-filled straws into the dough, alternating hands or using both hands as she does this. If the child is using ice cubes, have her pick them up using a single layer of thin cotton or waxed paper to reduce the chill.

Safety considerations: Limit the child's exposure to ice straws to a few seconds at a time.

Sensory considerations: If this is too challenging, have the child use an additional layer of cotton when picking up the ice filled straws or ice straws.

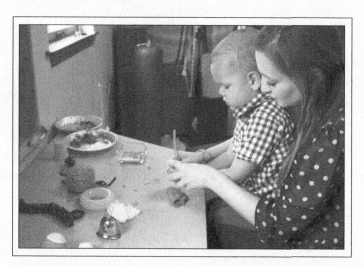

**Straws were filled with water, sealed with wax and put
in the freezer for an hour prior to this exercise.**

Easier Activities:

- Instead of ice straws, push unsharpened pencils into dough.
- Wrap ice cubes inside a thin dish towel and have the child hold them for a few seconds.
- Hold ice straws in the hand for five seconds.

Harder Activities:

- Take an ice cube from a tray and put it into a glass of water.
- Have the child bury seeds or stones deep and firmly into a pot of soil or in an outside garden area.

Walking a Plank - Plus

Activity: Walk on a 2 × 8-inch × 5-foot plank while carrying a chilled tray

Goals: To increase the ability to balance; improve attention and focus skills; integrate vision and motor.

Materials: A metal or plastic tray placed in the refrigerator; a board approximately two inches (5 centimeters) thick, eight inches (20 centimeters) wide, and minimally five feet (1.5 meters) long.

Instructions: Place the wooden plank on the floor near a wall so that the child can use it for support. Give the child a cooled tray and ask him to hold it as he walks back and forth on the plank.

Safety considerations: Touch the tray to ensure that it is not overly cold. To avoid a twisted ankle during a fall, the board should not be more than 2″ thick.

Sensory considerations: If the child has balance (vestibular) problems, remind her to lean on the wall for support, as needed.

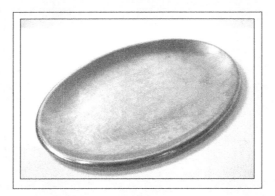

Carry tray while walking on the plank.

Easier Activities:

• Enrichments 4 and 11.

Harder Activities:

• Use a four-inch-wide (10 centimeter) board as a greater challenge for an older child.

Visual Attention to Massage

Activity: Rub fingers and toes in turn, while the child watches

Goals: To integrate visual and tactile senses; to increase touch sensory awareness.

Materials: None.

Instructions: Rub each of the child's fingers and toes as she looks on. Do this slowly over a 3-minute period.

Safety considerations: None.

Sensory considerations: None.

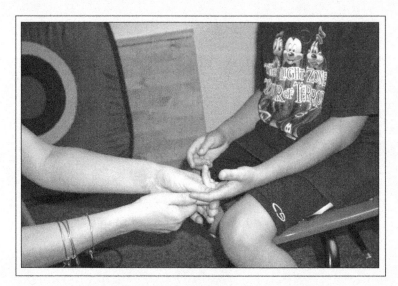

Therapist is giving a boy a finger massage.

Coins in a Piggy Bank with Mirror

Activity: Place coins in a piggy bank using only a mirrored reflection of hands

Goals: To increase visual motor skills and cognitive strategies.

Materials: Piggy bank, coins, small-medium sized mirror; folder, cardboard box or other item that can be used to occlude the child's sight of his hands as he sits at the table and puts coins in the piggy bank. (See photo and construction details, below.)

Instructions: Place a piggy bank and coins on a table. Place a standing mirror (or prop up a hand-held mirror) at the back of the table. Occlude the child's sight of the piggy bank by placing a folder or box at the front of the table. Have him sit at the table and put coins in the bank using only the reflection in the mirror of his hand, the bank and the coins.

Safety considerations: Make sure the mirror is secure.

Sensory considerations: None.

The setup for this exercise can be constructed using a 3-fold science project display board and a small mirror.

Easier Activities:

- Try some of the harder activities in Enrichment 15.
- Put an empty container and several objects on the table. Blindfold the child and ask her to find the objects and put them in the container.
- Put figurines and small cars on a table on their sides. Blindfold the child and ask her to set them upright.
- Have her comb hair in the mirror.

Harder Activities:

- Zip a jacket without looking at the hands.
- Button without looking at the hands.
- Button a shirt button while looking in the mirror.

Magnetic Fishing Pole

Activity: Pick up small objects using a thin pole with a magnet attached

Goals: Increased visual motor skills.

Materials: Toy fishing rod with a magnet at the end, or a home-made fishing rod constructed using a pen or ruler, string and a magnet; ten or more colorful metal paper clips or other small metal objects.

Instructions: Scatter paper clips on the table. Give the child the "fishing" rod and ask him to use it to pick up the paper clips.

Safety considerations: Do not put the magnet near electronic equipment or credit cards.

Sensory considerations: None.

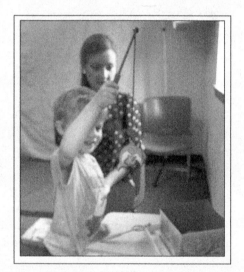 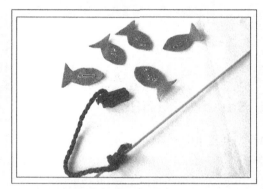

Games with magnetic fishing rods can be found in stores and online. However, you can make one using household materials and a small magnet.

Easier Activities:

• Give the child a ruler or small rod and ask him to use it to touch objects in the environment. The goal is to learn how to extend his reach using another object.

Harder Activities:

• Put small objects under a chair or dresser and ask the child to extract them ("fish them out") using a ruler.
• Put a shoe far under a bed and ask the child to recover it using a rod or a broom.

Visual Tracking

Activity: Track a red object as it moves around a picture

Goals: To increase visual tracking skills; to improve attention to task.

Materials: Pictures of well-known paintings. Find collections of pictures in used-book stores, the internet (search on "classical paintings for children"), or take photos at a museum.

Instructions: Put the picture on the table and let the child look at it for a few moments. Next, put the red object next to the photo and tell him, "Look at the red ____." Move the object slowly around the picture, telling him, "Keep looking."

Safety considerations: None.

Sensory considerations: If the child is colorblind, be sure to use a bright, preferably red, object.

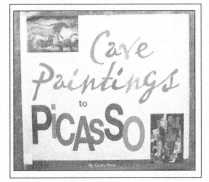

Books like Cave Paintings to Picasso by H. Sayre, are a good source of child-appropriate artwork through the ages.

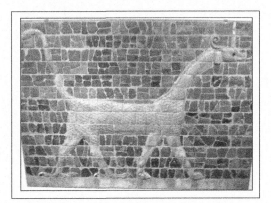

Photo of Mosaic: Marduk, god of Baal, Detroit Institute of Arts.

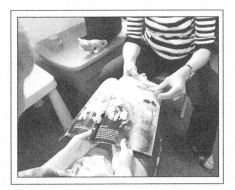

Therapist holds a large red bead and moves it around a picture of a dinosaur while the child tries to keep her eyes on the red bead.

Easier Activities:

- In a darkened room, use a flashlight to create clockwise and counter-clockwise circles on the wall. Ask the child to keep head still and her eye on the flashlight beam. Make the circles small enough for her to look at without moving her head.
- With a flashlight, slowly trace a large circle on the wall and ask the child to move her eyes, following the path of the light.

Harder Activities:

- Use a favorite picture for the background image (dinosaurs, trains, or cartoon characters) to increase the challenge for paying attention to task.
- Put an eye chart just above eye-level on a wall near a trampoline. As the child jumps, ask her to read a row or column of letters. You can make an eye chart on a large sheet of paper by neatly printing rows of numbers and letters in marker. Make sure the columns line up.

Navigating Stairway Without Hands

Activity: Walk up and down stairs while holding a big ball or pillow

Goals: To improve balance, attention and coordination; to integrate the vestibular and touch senses.

Materials: A big ball or a pillow; stairway.

Instructions: Give the child the ball or pillow and ask her to walk up and down the stairs.

Safety considerations: An adult should stay on the steps just below the child as she walks, in case she loses balance or slips.

Sensory considerations: Some children are afraid of steps due to poor vestibular function. Make a set of short steps using reams of paper, bricks or sturdy blocks. Have the child master this, then gradually increase the step height. For persistent problems, occupational therapy or physical therapy is recommended.

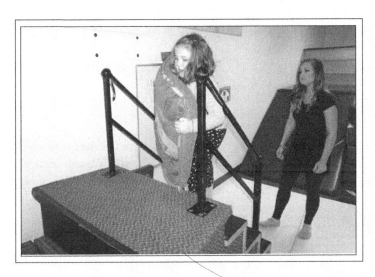

Child carries a bolster up a short staircase.

Easier Activities:

- Have the child carry a succession of soft objects up and down stairs while holding the rail. Start with small objects, and then move to bulkier items.
- Have the child walk up and down stairs without holding the rail and with nothing in his hands.

Harder Activities:

- Continue this activity with larger and heavier items. Have an older child carry a laundry basket, book bag or stack of games up and down stairs.

Draw What You Feel

Activity: Draw shapes using pencil and paper to match shapes being drawn on the child's back (over shirt)

Goals: To increase visual-motor skills; to integrate touch, vision and motor; to learn to ignore distracting and conflicting sensory input.

Materials: Paper and pencil or fat crayon; one or more toys that can be used to draw with.

Instructions: Put a pen and paper on the table. Have the child draw a shape. As she does, draw the same shape on her back using your finger. Switch up. Draw a shape on the child's back and have her copy what she senses onto paper. Continue taking turns.

Safety considerations: If the child mouths objects, be sure to use non-toxic drawing materials.

Sensory considerations: If the child is tactile defensive (dislikes being touched), the adult should press firmly while drawing. Also consider providing calming input to the child such as a back massage or shoulder squeezes before drawing on her back. Also, see the *sensory consideration* section of Enrichment 1 for additional ideas.

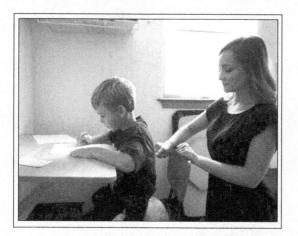

The therapist draws shapes on the child's back while he senses the shape and then draws it.

Easier Activities:

- Teach the child to draw lines and shapes.
- Draw only lines, circles or dots on the child's back and ask him to guess what you have drawn.
- Add new shapes, one at a time, until the child is proficient at registering and then drawing them.

Harder Activities:

- Tell her to draw a shape like a triangle, circle, or square on paper while you draw a different shape on her back.
- Talk about what the shapes can be used for in a drawing. For example, when you draw a triangle, ask, "What part of a house is this? Continue by drawing other parts of a house on her back such as a square for the main part of the house, a rectangle for the door, and so on, all the while guiding her to draw a house with all of it parts.
- Ask her to name the shape you've drawn and tell you what objects are shaped that way.

Enrichment 30

Draw with Two Hands

Activity: Draw lines on paper using both hands simultaneously

Goals: To increase bimanual skills and overall right brain and left brain integration of a motor movement.

Materials: Paper; two fat crayons, pens or pencils.

Instructions: Ask the child to pick up a pencil in each hand. If he is young, place his hands so that the pencil tips are touching the top of the page. Tell him to draw lines, using both pencils and both hands, from the top of the page to the bottom. Have him draw other lines, again using both pencils and both hands, from one side to the other and from the lower edge of the paper to the top, and so on.

Safety considerations: If the child mouths objects, use non-toxic markers instead of pencils.

Sensory considerations: You may need to help the child hold the pencil correctly. A fisted grip is appropriate for young children. The grip will slowly mature to a standard pencil grasp around the age of five or six. It is important not to force a mature grasp on a young child.

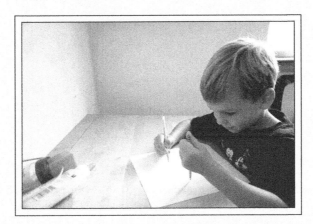

Boy is drawing lines simultaneously with both hands.

Easier Activities:

- Do the activity with your hands over the child's hands, until he gets the hang of it.
- Have the child hold a pencil in his non-dominant hand and use the dominant hand guide it in drawing a line.
- Have the child draw in the air with his index fingers, moving both fingers simultaneously, for 5-10 seconds.
- Have the child draw lines and circles in the air with both fingers together.
- Try the previous exercises with fingers moving on or just above the table.

Harder Activities:

- Begin simple bimanual activities such as closing snaps, and pulling Velcro™ apart.
- Continue with harder bimanual activities such as buttoning, lacing cards, snipping with scissors, and zipping.

Match Colors

Activity: Match colored beads to the colors of objects in a photo

Goals: To increase visual motor skills; to increase visual awareness and attention to task.

Materials: Photos of objects (use picture books, or photos you have taken); a container with colored beads.

Instructions: Place colored pictures and colored beads on the table. Have the child match the colors in the photos with the beads.

Safety considerations: None.

Sensory considerations: Be alert for signs of color blindness.

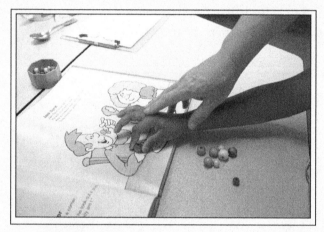

Child selects a bead to match the color of the man's shirt.

Easier Activities:

- Enrichments 10, 12, 20 and their alternate activities.
- Put small pieces of different colored papers on the table and match beads to the pieces of paper.

Harder Activities:

- Draw simple shapes (circles, squares, and triangles) on small cardstock. One shape per card. Pick one of the shapes and look for that shape in picture books. Keep this simple at first by using books with shapes as the subject.
- Repeat the previous exercise with picture books showing objects with shapes you have been working with. For example, ask the child to find the circles in a picture of a bicycle.

Blow Foil or Feather

Activity: Blow aluminum foil or a small feather on the floor as far as possible

Goals: To integrate (oral) motor skills with visual skills. In addition, blowing activates facial and respiratory muscles which are used to display emotions and to regulate breathing.

Materials: Small pieces of aluminum foil or feathers.

Instructions: Place a small piece of aluminum foil on the floor. Have the child lie on the floor and blow the foil as far as possible. Once he gets the hang of this, place small targets on the floor and ask him to try to hit the targets.

Safety considerations: None.

Sensory considerations: None.

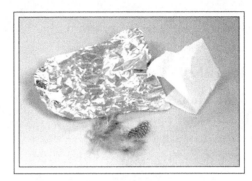

Foil, paper, a feather

Easier Activities:

- If the child does not yet know how to blow, try these procedures:
  o Have the child observe you and imitate your mouth movement. Gently form his mouth into an O shape, and tell him to blow. Use a mirror for this activity.
  o Blow bubbles with bubble soap as a way of increasing motivation. Put the soap in a bowl to make it easier. You blow first, then ask him to blow. Gently plug his nose to send air out of his mouth.

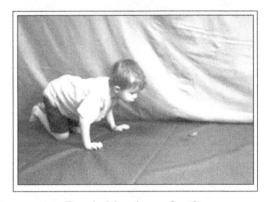

Boy is blowing a feather across the floor

Harder Activities:

- Keep a balloon in the air using the breath only.
- See the additional exercises in Chapter 5 that make use of whistles and kazoos.

Visual Attention with Moving Pictures

Activity: View two pictures as they repeatedly move from back to front and back again

Goals: To increase attention to task; to help the child move between (and be aware of) different visual frames-of-reference.

Materials: Two or more pictures.

Instructions: With a photo in each hand, present the photos to the child, with one in front of the other. Talk about the picture, if only to say, "Here are two pictures, here is the first picture." Then move the front picture to the back and the back one to the front, and say, "Here is the second picture." With time, name elements in the pictures as they alternate moving into view, and also prompt the child to say something about each picture, "That's grandma, that's a cat." Make a game of it.

Safety considerations: None.

Sensory considerations: None.

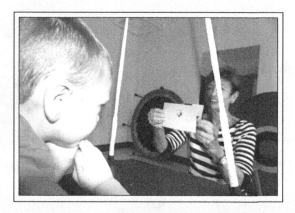

**Boy attends to back-to-back pictures, telling his therapist
what he sees in each picture as she brings one, then the other into view.**

Easier Activities:

• Enrichments 13, 27 and their alternate activities.
• Enrichment 17 and its alternate activities.

Harder Activities:

• Ask the child to say what he sees each time the picture is swapped.
• Give the child a book with different images on each page, such as an alphabet book for small children or an age-appropriate picture book for older children. Tell the child that you are going to look at each page and say what you see. Go through 5-10 pages.
• Have the child turn the pages and name what he sees.

Pictures and Music

Activity: Listen to music that corresponds to a photo

Goals: To integrate hearing and vision; to integrate the senses with cognitive processing.

Materials: Songs and music albums with a theme such as ethnic music; photos in a book or on the internet that are associated with the music. Take the opportunity in this exercise to introduce the child to new sensory and cultural input, but also include child-friendly themes such as trains and theme parks and familiar activities such as brushing teeth.

Instructions: Play some music, and then show pictures that are related to the music. In a few words, describe the connection. For example, "This is music from Ireland. Here is a picture of the island of Ireland. Here is a picture of houses in Ireland," and so on.

Safety considerations: None.

Sensory considerations: Allow the child to select (and to reject) some percentage of the music, but attempt to acclimate her to both music as a whole and to different styles of it.

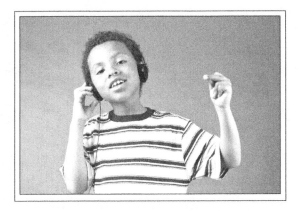

Have the child listen and move (dance) to music from around the world. Dancing will help with rhythm entrainment and help decrease undesirable behaviors associated with sound. Start slowly with music that is similar to what she currently likes. Avoid playing more than a minute or two of music that she finds annoying.

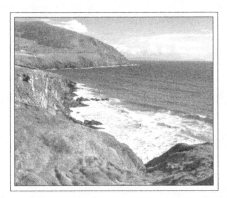

A picture of the island of Ireland

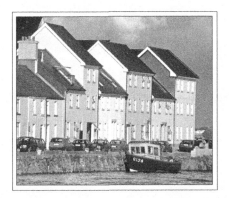

A picture of houses in Ireland

CHAPTER 5

Enrichment Mix-Ins

Here are additional enrichment exercises to build foundation skills for children with autism and special needs. The activities involve speech, emotional awareness, facial affect, verbal rhythm, motor rhythm and basic movement. These important skill areas are not covered in the Environmental Enrichment Protocol.

The speech and emotion activities are designed to encourage expressive communication. They include reading books together, playing simple instruments and doing activities that make noise. The motor activities were selected to increase functional and novel movement, and to enhance the child's sense of motor rhythm.

Most of the mix-ins are fun and can be added into the Environmental Enrichment exercise sessions as an interlude or offered at the end as a reward for completing the activities. They do not replace the original set of exercises.

Mix-in Enrichment 1

Toot a Whistle

Goals: To activate facial muscles for the purpose of producing facial expression and productive speech; to increase imitation skills.

Materials: Two simple whistles; optionally a mirror.

Instructions: Have the child blow into the whistle until he makes a sound. Focus on producing a clean sound. Each of you can blow a whistle together in the mirror so that he can see what you do.

Safety considerations: For a young child, avoid small whistles that can be choking hazards.

Sensory considerations: If the child is generally sensitive to sound, play softly and from a distance as you demonstrate the instrument or create a video of playing it, and play back the video with reduced sound. She will probably be able to tolerate the sound of her own tooting.

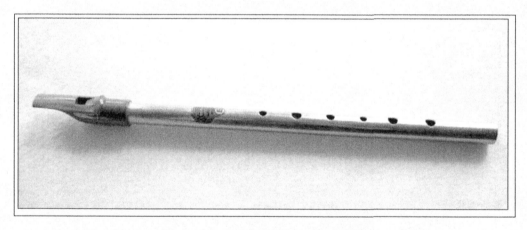

Therapeutic whistles are rated from beginner on up.
But try any appropriate whistle you might have on hand, like this penny whistle.

Blow a Horn, Toot a Whistle

Goals: To activate facial muscles as an aid to speaking, intonation and expressing emotions.

Materials: Kazoo, penny whistle, small horn, harmonica and other mouth instruments.

Instructions: Have the child blow into the whistle until he makes a sound. Focus on producing a clean sound. Once that is mastered, try to produce different tones and short sequences of tones. For the kazoo, instruct the child to make a sound as he blows into it. If you are using an instrument that requires finger placement, such as the penny whistle, cover a hole for the child as he blows, and then show him how to do it.

Safety considerations: None.

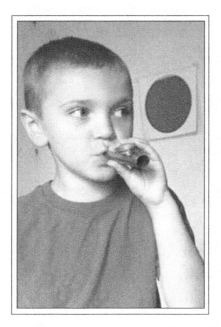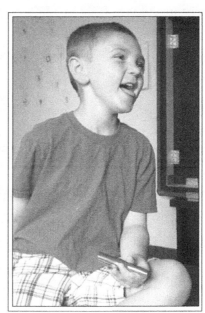

Boy having fun humming into a kazoo.

Sensory considerations: If the child is generally sensitive to sound, demonstrate the instrument softly from a distance. When it is her turn to play, she will probably find her own tooting less irritating. If she continues to experience sensitivity, create a video of you playing the instrument and then play it for her throughout the day with reduced sound.

Make Animal Sounds

Use this for the child who has few verbal skills.

Goals: To learn to make animal sounds.

Materials: Optional: animal pictures or books; small animal toys.

Instructions: Do one or more of the following

1. Look at pictures of animals and make the appropriate sound. Have the child repeat it.

2. Sing "Old MacDonald" and have the child help with the animal sounds (or the entire song).

3. Together, make other animal sounds such as snorting, yipping and hissing.

Safety considerations: None.

Sensory considerations: None.

Easy Animal Sounds

Baa-aa

Moo-oo

Me-ow-w

Ruff-ruff

Nei-eigh

Quack, quack

Practice B and P Words

"B" and "p" are early sounds and make a good starter exercise for the non-verbal child.

Goals: To learn to say "b" and "p" sounds.

Materials: Pictures in books or online of the words starting with "b" and "p".

Instructions: In these exercises, the focus is on the initial "bah" and "pah" sounds rather than on saying the entire word. Feel free to add additional simple words to these lists.

B and P Words

Ball, bubbles, baby, ball, bull, bear, bug, blue, button, bag, big, backpack
Puppy, pig, peach, panda, paper, paw, pink, purple,hippo, apple,
pie, pot, pan, penguin

---

1. Show a picture of a "b" or "p" word from the list, and then say it, emphasizing the "bah" or "pah" sound. Ask the child to say it with you.

2. Once she can say the words with you, show her the picture and ask her what it is. Help her, if necessary, by slowly sounding the word and exaggerating your mouth movement.

3. Ask the child to say the initial "b" and "p" words in these simple sentences and phrases.

   a. The baby plays.   g. Beat on the pot.
   b. The pig is pink.   h. I have a big, purple plum.
   c. The puppy likes bubbles.   i. Peel the potato.
   d. The bear has a blue ball.   j. Pam is pretty.
   e. The boy watches a bug.   k. Buddy baked a pie.
   f. The bear has brown paws.

4. Nonsense phrases are fun for the older child. Say them slowly, then quickly, and repeat. Feel free to make up your own nonsense phrases.
   a. Be bop bim
   b. Bubba baby booboo
   c. Peppy pepper pie
   d. Potato popup patty
   e. Bat paw pal pod

Safety considerations: None.

Sensory considerations: None.

Teaching Gestures

It's equally important for children to be able to sign or gesture back to their parents. Practical signing commands include "more," "stop," "all done," "water," "eat," "pain" (or medicine), and "help." Also include the toileting signs, "change" (diaper) or "bathroom".

As you teach a sign, recite the word singly or in a short phrase: "stop," or "I want water."

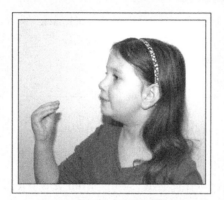 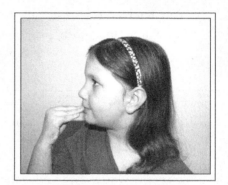

Eat: Move the hand as if stuffing food into the mouth.

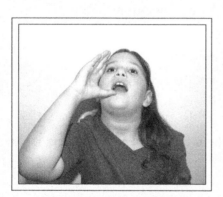 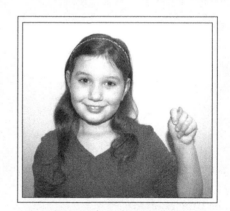

Drink

Bathroom: Shake the hand back and forth (or twist it) as you make the sign for "t".

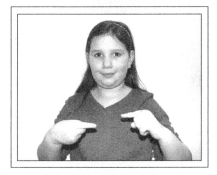 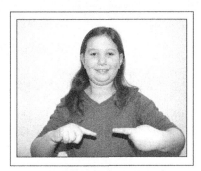

Hurt, pain: Twist the hands back and forth as you make the sign. Point to the place that hurts. Use facial expression, the more it hurts, the bigger the expression.

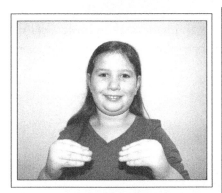 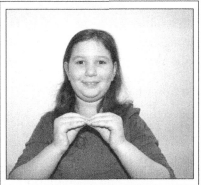

More: Move hands together and then let them bounce in place.

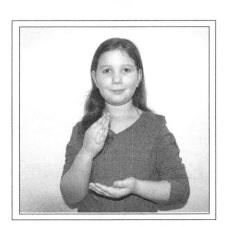 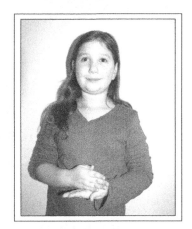

Stop

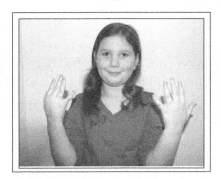

Finished, or all done

Mix-in Enrichment 6

Make Faces in the Mirror

Children with autism have difficulty both in expressing emotion and in recognizing it in others. Here is a simple set of exercises to engage the key facial muscles used for emotions. As you try each one in the mirror, compare your face to the child's and help her with the subtleties of face muscle movement. Some people can feel emotion as it triggers the heart. By tapping on your heart as you say the emotion, you encourage the child to sense that internal sensation.

Goals: To activate facial muscles and to integrate that sensation with recognition of emotions.

Materials: A mirror.

Instructions: While standing with the child in front of a mirror, make simple faces using the techniques below. Before assuming each face, say the name of the emotion. Tap on your heart as you say the emotion and say "I see [emotion] on my face. I feel it in my heart. Look at this!"

1. Pencil between lips – happy
2. Pencil between teeth – mad
3. Teeth on inner curled lip – disgust
4. Cheek muscles up, lips out – sad
5. Eyebrows up, lips curled down – unhappy
6. Smile with "cheese" – very happy, excited
7. Lower lip curled – pout

Safety considerations: None.

Sensory considerations: None.

Mix-in Enrichment 7

Name an Emotion

Goals: To activate facial muscles and to integrate that sensation with recognition of emotions.

Materials: Your hand drawn faces; commercial products such as Kimochi™ Mixed Feelings; books illustrating emotions such as *How Are You Peeling*; pictures of emotional faces; and emoticon apps.

Instructions:

1. Display an exaggerated emotion on your face. Tell the child to look at your face. Ask him, "What am I feeling?" Give him clues and possible answers to choose from, "Am I tired or excited?"
2. Show pictures and drawings of faces from sources listed in the materials list. Ask him to name the emotion. Then ask him to put that emotion on his face.
3. Ask the older child to draw cartoon figures with emotional faces. If this is fun for him, use cartooning as a way of exploring facial emotions.

Mix-in Enrichment 8

Running in Place or Fast Marching to a Beat

Goals: To increase rhythm skills; to increase lower-body coordination skills.

Materials: None.

Instructions: Start with a rhythmic march-in-place movement and then increase the speed to a slow run (in-place). Do this for 20 seconds. With time, continue to increase the speed and have the child raise her knees higher.

Safety considerations: Be aware of child's balance skills.

Sensory considerations: None.

Mix-in Enrichment 9

Beat a Drum

Learning to recognize and keep a beat helps our internal brain rhythms.

Goals: To learn rhythms; to provide rhythmic input to the brain's processing circuitry for internal synchronization.

Materials: Table top, oatmeal box, small drum or bongo.

Instructions: Tap out simple rhythms such as those below and ask the child to do what you do.

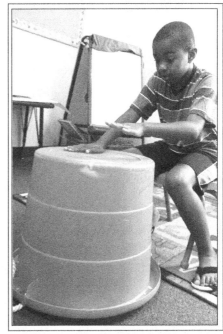

1. Steady tapping on drum with one hand.
2. Steady tapping with both hands.
3. Steady tapping with alternating hands.
4. Two taps with left hand then two taps with right while keeping a steady beat.

Boy beating a makeshift drum.

Mix-in Enrichment 10

Basic Exercise Movements

These basic movements are a good foundation for learning to exercise and to play on play equipment. Young children should be able to do the simple movements. A school-aged child can typically do all of these, including jumping jacks.

Goals: To learn the basic movements needed for exercise and play.

Materials: None.

Instructions: Perform one or more of these steps for ten seconds each. Between steps, take a 5-10 second rest break.

1. Jump in place.
2. Jump up, then come down with legs apart (this is the legs portion of jumping jacks).
3. Downward dog
4. Superman
5. Roll up
6. Climbing onto stool
7. Shimmy

Safety considerations: If the child struggles with balance, position her near a wall.

Sensory considerations: None.

Jumping

Practice jumping in a variety of ways: a simple jump up; a jump high in the air with arms swinging up to help achieve the height; and a long jump.

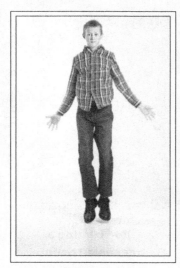

A simple jump

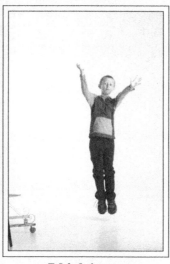

A high jump

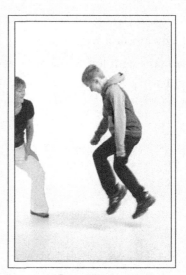

Long jump

Simple Half-Jumping Jacks

Children with special needs may struggle to perform the coordinated movements of jumping jacks. You can help the child learn the parts by breaking down the complex jumping jack moves into simpler steps. Try these alternate methods. Here are three easy exercises to help the child learn the individual arm and leg movements. Practice all three with the child, and then try a few "real" jumping jacks to see how she is progressing.

Arms up in a clap, then down to the side

The easiest portion of jumping jacks is the arm movement. Tell the child to clap his arms above the head and then bring them back down to the side. Do several in a row. Work with the chid to achieve a clean symmetric movement with arms straight out and moving together.

Arms out, legs apart in a star

Have the child place his arms to the side, and his legs apart (in a star position). Then move back to standing position. Once he can do that successfully, practice jumping into the star position and back: jump and land with legs apart and arms out to the side, and then jump back. Practice this until his movements are smooth.

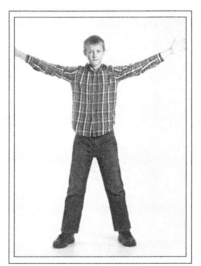 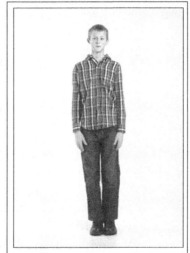

Right side, back to center, left side

In this variation, the child swings one arm and leg up, then returns to arms down and legs together. Do each side separately, and then alternate.

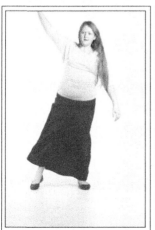 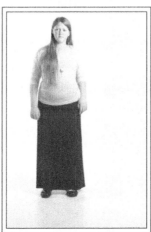 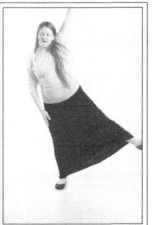 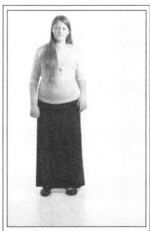

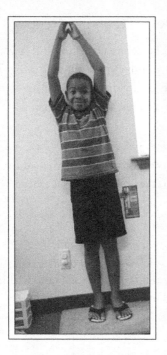

Extension and Flexion

It is important for our extension and flexion muscles to be strong because they support each other in movement. Here are simple exercises that help the child stretch and strengthen those muscle sets.

Downward dog

A very young child can do downward dog. As the child matures, help her learn to extend her muscles completely and form her body into a perfect inverted "V" position. An older child should be able to hold the pose for eight seconds with ease.

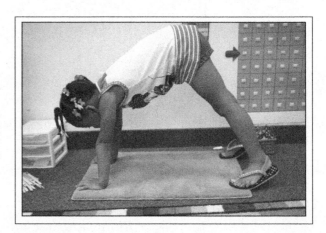

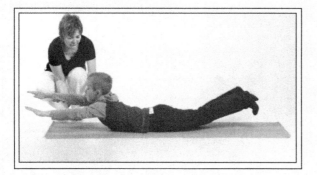

Superman

Superman is a good exercise for strengthening the core muscles. Encourage the child to hold the position for 20-30 seconds. If that is difficult, practice the stretch until he can.

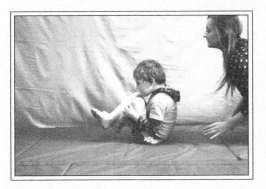 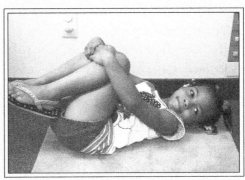

Flexion (Roll-up)

A five-year-old can easily do this, but you may need to remind a four-year-old to tuck her head in. Hold the flexed position for eight seconds, and then over time slowly increase it to 25-30 seconds.

Step Up

Climbing skills are essential play skills for children. If the child with autism is unable to climb, a visit to an occupational or physical therapist is in order. This next exercise builds on climbing skills as we literally take the child to the next step in climbing movement by having the child safely step up onto a stool or chair and then back down.

Big step up

Select a chair that is knee height or shorter for the child to step on. Place it on a non-slip surface next to a wall. Step up five times with the right foot. *Encourage the child to place his hand on the wall for support.* Repeat this exercise with the left foot. When the child is able to step up and down smoothly, alternate the starting foot with each step up. Do 10 step-ups and step-downs, alternating feet.

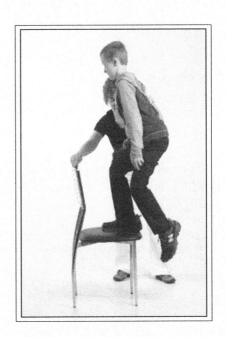

Cross Midline

The challenge in this next exercise is to cross midline—a skill that develops around age three or four, but is quite difficult for many children with special needs. We start with a shimmy. We'll continue with an *almost-touch opposite toes* exercise at the end of this section.

Shimmy side-to-side

The shimmy can be broken into two parts: 1) twisting from side to side, and 2) wiggling while moving up and down. Practice each of these separately and then perform the whole shimmy.

Shimmy: simultaneously twist from side-to-side and move up and down while keeping the neck and head faced forward. The arms should move across midline. Help the child move his hands across midline until he is able to motor-plan that action on his own. Do this for 10 seconds.

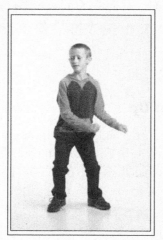 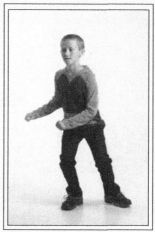

More Exercises

Finally, we get to the pre-cursors of pushups, toe touches, windmills and step-ups. Here are easier versions of those exercises.

Knee push-ups

Push-ups help a child to maintain good core strength. While an older child with typical motor skills should be able to do full push-ups, a 5-6 year-old will find it easier to do knee push-ups. Knee push-ups are a good place to start with children with autism. Do a few and try to increase the number each time. You may need to help position the child for this exercise. You may also need to help him pull up his body weight by pulling up on his shoulders or chest as he pushes up. Slowly let him assume the full job, with time.

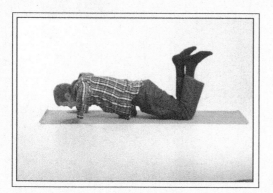 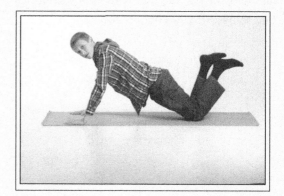

Almost-touch toes

Touching toes is a good way to stretch. The exercise helps to pull energy out of wiggly muscles. In this easier version, we want the child to focus on stretching as far as she can—to almost touch her toes. Do five toe-touches, *slowly*. Encourage the child to reach just a little further each time.

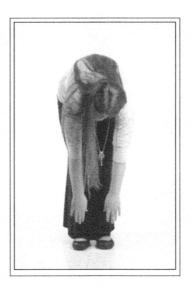

Almost-touch opposite toes (half-windmills)

This exercise is a precursor to learning windmills: "almost touch" the opposite toe.

Help the child move her hands and twist her body across midline until she is able to motor-plan that action on her own. As with touching toes, it is more important, when doing the exercise, to get the stretch than to force the reach to the toes. Do 10 touches, alternating each side. See if the child can reach just a little further with each alternation.

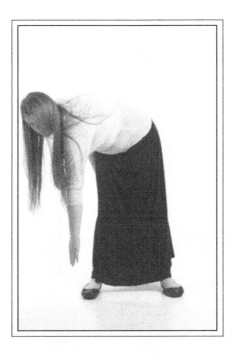
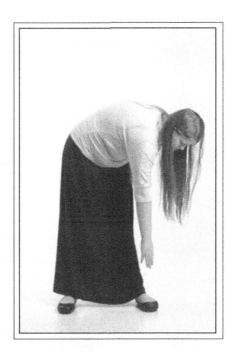

Section III

SENSORY ENRICHMENT ACTIVITIES

In this section of the book, we look at fun activities for sensory desensitization and sensory immersion. We use *desensitization* techniques to slowly acclimate a child to sensations that irritate him such as loud noises, a light touch on the skin or the taste of food. We use *immersion techniques* to give a child enough sensory input to help an undersensitive child register input, satisfy the need for sensation in a child who craves it, and provide pleasant, calming input for the oversensitive child.

The desensitization techniques and some of the immersion techniques can be used as an extension of the environmental enrichment program. The remaining immersion activities such as working with fibers and wood are stand-alone activities that can help provide a child with specific sensations while teaching him basic skills useful for a hobby.

You can use immersion and desensitization activities:

1. As an extension to the environmental enrichment program or a maintenance program for it.

2. As a way to help sensitize children to sensory input so that they are able to handle the sensory demands of their day.

3. As a way to satiate the desire for sensory input in a child who craves it.

4. As a way to wake up the senses in a child who is undersensitive to sensory input.

5. As ideas for providing informal daily exposure to sensory input for all children.

6. As a source for activities within a sensory diet.

Immersion and Desensitization Activities

The next chapters of this section contain a range of immersion strategies for each of the senses. As in the environmental enrichment program, exercises and activities are graded by difficulty. Given that each child's preferences for materials and activity type will differ, a number of approaches are presented for each sense in this section. Once you see the types of immersion activities offered for a particular sense, you will realize you can extrapolate from there and come up with your own ideas.

Who initiates these activities and when? Caregivers, educators and therapists will find these activities useful. Most exercises can be fit into a normal day and repeated as desired. The multiday, multi-sensory projects in chapter 11 can be slowly completed over a week or two.

How much time do I spend? That will depend on the child and upon your opportunities.

Immersion for craving and sensitization

We use sensory immersion techniques for children who crave certain types of sensory input or for children who have trouble feeling and registering sensation. Look for immersion activities that will provide a large quantity of sustained input. With touch, for example, you might engage the child in multi-day craft projects that provide strong input while producing an interesting object.

How much: Immerse the child in sensations he craves by giving him sense-specific activities for 15-30 minutes at a time, or until he appears to have had enough.

How often: Engage the child two or more times per week. An immersion activity can be considered to be the child's "sensory break." If it is calming, alerting and interesting to the child, it can help to reduce stress and increase motivation to engage in the next task. Use immersion activities also with children with autism who "stim."

At what level of challenge: Consider working up to long projects that give the child:

1. A sense of rhythm with a constant activity

2. An activity that can be converted into a hobby

3. The satisfaction of creating something tangible

Other instructions: If you are working with multiple senses, look for multi-sensory activities. Optionally, rotate through sense-specific activities (i.e. bead a bracelet, listen to music) two or more times each week.

How do I select immersion activities? Immersion activities are chosen, first to satisfy sensory needs (both craving and poor registration) and, second to teach children new skills and hobbies that can be used to enrich their lives and, perhaps, their adult lives, too. For example, Aaron, who sniffs objects, might enjoy cooking, gardening or other activities that expose him to a rich set of odors and aromas. In turn, this might lead to a job as a florist or a cook or to a cooking hobby. Sabrina, who constantly touches things, might enjoy activities with wood, metal, clay or fabric.

A note about working with multiple senses: When doing immersion, make every intervention count by looking for simple ways to increase the essential sensory content. For example, Ben, who has autism, likes to touch things and also "stims on" visual input. We might give Ben daily touch activities that also stimulate him visually, thus working on two problems simultaneously.

When multiple types of sensory input are given to the child within the same activity, the child's brain is able to integrate the interaction of those senses. That is, his brain will practice recognizing and tolerating each input simultaneously—and then in tandem. However, it is important that we do not overload and overwhelm the child's sensory system with too much input. We try and give the child the just-right challenge. This important point is discussed in chapter 1.

A note about craving: Sensory craving is a common phenomenon in children with autism. A child may enjoy touching things that have interesting textures such as a fuzzy toy, another child's hair, or the feel of cloth. He may enjoy the sound, sparkle and feel of water. Some children with autism wave their hands under a running faucet in the sink and fuss when they are asked to stop. Other children may enjoy sniffing things of all sorts and often do it inappropriately.

There are several strategies for working with cravings. The most straightforward method, when it works, is to allow the child to engage in a socially appropriate form of the behavior for a short period of time. Manage this by setting a timer—usually a visual timer—for 5-10 minutes. The child learns that when his time is up he must move on to other activities.

Desensitization

Desensitization is difficult work for the child. Look for activities that are fun and make it easier for her to shore up courage.

How much: Do however much the child can tolerate at a time. This may be just a minute or two with attention.

At what level of challenge: Grade the challenge so that the child can tolerate the input, but then gradually increase the level of input.

How often: In most cases, three times a day is not too much. At a minimum, do the activities three times a week.

Other instructions: Do a calming activity such as exhaustive play or, for older children, mindfulness. This may allow the child to tolerate longer and greater amounts of the sensory input. But honor the child's limits.

The safest way to get started with desensitization is to introduce new sensations during play. We begin by giving the child small amounts of input and then gradually increasing the input as he is able to handle it. When possible, we give the child some control during these activities. This helps ensure that the pace is right for the child and it reduces the incidence of act-out behaviors. In addition, we provide calming techniques to help him stay regulated and keep fear under control.

To make a program:

1. Set up a daily or weekly schedule

2. Plan activities

3. Plan how you will increase the challenge

4. Stick to the plan

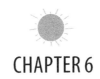

CHAPTER 6

Touch

Touch Desensitizing

Here is a set of activities, listed in order of difficulty, to help a child desensitize to gooey materials. These activities make use of glues and doughs which are easily found materials. As the child progresses in ability to touch glue and dough, think of slowly incorporating gooey foods (yogurt and bananas), and toiletries (shampoos and lotions) into her day.

Go slow with each activity. Let the child be your guide as you decide how much to do in a day. Don't worry that you didn't do enough. Even a few minutes of exposure can be useful. Make sure to do a small activity at least 3-4 days a week so that the progress made "sticks." Remember that a calming activity prior to "facing the gooey stuff" can make your job easier.

It's wise to have a small cup of water and a small towel nearby to get the goo off fingertips immediately before the child becomes overwhelmed.

Activities to avoid

Avoid finger painting, vegetable printing and other activities that make use of washable paints, food coloring and inks. Most washable paints are hard to wash off and leave a residue of color. The sight of this could potentially cause alarm. Instead, allow the child to use a brush for painting and keep soapy water and a towel nearby.

A note about touch sensitivities and autism

Children with autism as a group are known to have mild-to-severe sound and touch sensitivities. The underlying problem appears to be different than typical oversensitivity. In children with autism, the boundaries between sense regions (touch, vision, auditory) appear to be blurred. In addition, the connectors between regions are thicker than in children without autism. As a result, they struggle to process and interpret the touch (and other sense) input they receive.

In some cases, signals aren't modulated. Some children with autism feel pain when touched on the head during shampooing or hair combing, as well as when their nails are clipped. Desensitizing a child to touch and pain in this instance is tricky. One solution is to thoroughly prepare the child through calming and setting expectations. Another solution is to give the child control over the task (hair combing, for example) and let him do it himself. I cover additional strategies for working with these issues in my book, *Self-Regulation Interventions and Strategies*.

These activities in later chapters also have touch input:

Food activity, Ch. 7	Scent activity, Ch. 7	Vision activity, Ch. 9
#3, Drawing with food	#6, Scented dough	#2, Fabric swatches
		#11, Scented-fruit mobile
		#13, Collage with dried flowers

Cut-and-Paste with a Glue Stick

Materials: Glue sticks; all kinds of paper; magazine pages; small cup of water and a small towel.

We start touch desensitization with a glue-stick activity. Most children with touch sensitivities tolerate using a glue stick, and so this is an easy place to start. However, they are still sticky, and so should be introduced matter-of-factly, and used just for a quick cut-and-paste activity. Keep a paper towel at hand. If there appears to be resistance, keep activities brief and slowly work up to harder tasks such as folding a sheet in two and gluing it together.

Cut-and-Paste with School Glue and a Brush

Materials: A small cup with a mixture of school glue and water; a brush; colored paper, scissors; a small cup of water and a paper towel; optional: decorative materials such as stones or glitter.

Instructions: Set out paper and scissors for a cut-and-paste activity. In a small cup, mix a small amount of water into some school glue. Have the child brush the glue onto the paper, and carefully place the cut-out on top. Remind him that he can wash off any glue that gets on his fingers. Optionally, create by gluing small stones to paper or work with glitter glue instead. The thinned glue mixture will need longer to dry.

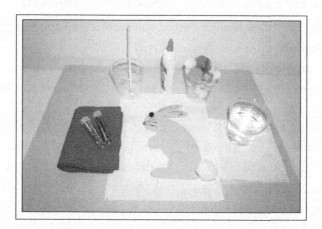

Use brushes and applicators for spreading glue during the initial stages of the desensitization process. Keep water and a paper towel handy.

School Glue and a Bunny Tail

A small child can enjoy the sensations of pom-poms and glitter as he learns to tolerate gooey substances. Here is a simple exposure to using school glue that includes soft, calming-to-the-touch pompoms.

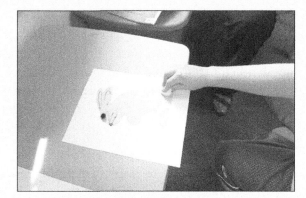

The pleasant sensation of a pompom cottontail overrides the displeasure of having to get fingers close to glue.

Materials: Construction paper; pompoms for the eye and tail; school glue; glitter or glitter glue for the whiskers and ears; image of bunny (in the Appendix); small cup of water and a small towel; optional: scrap of red felt, buttons, beans and stones.

1. Set a cup of water and towel on the table. Put a bit of school glue in a small cup. Optionally, mix it with a few drops of water to make it less sticky.
2. Make a copy of the bunny and cut it out, and glue it to a sheet of paper using a brush.
3. Use the bottle of school glue to apply glue for the eye and tail pompoms.
4. The nose can be made using a scrap of construction paper or felt. Have the child brush glue on the bunny's nose and use his fingers to put the nose in place. If he hesitates, remind him there is water nearby to wash glue off his fingers—or offer to put the nose in place for him.
5. Make whiskers and the inside ear detail using glitter glue or glue and sprinkled glitter.
6. Draw extra details as desired.

Make Collages with Paper Using a Glue Stick, Then School Glue

Create a collage from found pictures, cut-outs, and small objects like pebbles or leaves. Use a combination of gluing methods: glue stick, glue and brush and school glue in a bottle depending on the size and shape of the object to be glued. Keep a paper towel nearby to wipe glue off fingers.

Materials: Cardstock or heavy paper; different color papers including papers with print, giftwrap and pages from magazine; school glue; scissors; markers or crayons; a cup of water and a small towel; optional: found objects such as small beads, pebbles, flower petals, leaves, and so on.

1. Set out the cup of water and towel.
2. Cut pictures and text from magazines or shapes from colored and printed paper.
3. Arrange them and any found objects you are using on a piece of cardstock or heavy paper and, one by one, glue them in place.
4. Complete the collage by decorating with crayons or markers.

Make Mosaics with Glue Stick and School Glue

Mosaics are a fun project for children of all ages. The challenge for the child lies in gluing small bits of paper in place. There is a good possibility that the child will accidently touch the glue—and touch it often. So keep the atmosphere calm. Most important, do just a little at a time, stopping when the child has had enough. This project can be done over a period of several days or longer.

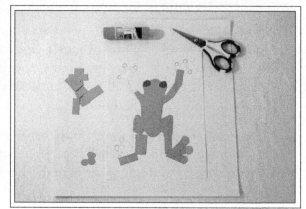

Let a child get used to the sensation of glue-from a glue stick prior to having him work with school glue.

Materials: Cardstock or heavy paper; different color papers; one of more large shapes for the mosaic; school glue; scissors or paper cutter; a cup of water and a small towel. Use very simple shapes or pictures such as a heart, a house with trees or the tree frog (in the Appendix). An older child might try a more detailed picture.

Instructions:

1. Set out the cup of water and towel.

2. Draw a simple picture onto the cardstock or lightly glue a coloring book page to it.

3. You can create the "tiles" in one of two ways:

   a. Cut up small or medium size pieces of colored paper to use as tiles in the mosaic.

   b. Copy the main shapes of the picture onto appropriately colored paper. Cut out the shapes, then cut them into smaller, but recognizable, pieces—like a jigsaw puzzle—to be glued onto paper. See the picture of the tree frog, above.

4. Put a small amount of glue in place, and then place one or more squares onto the drawing. Keep the water and towel handy for when she touches the glue.

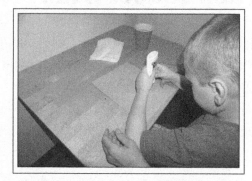

To make a quick mosaic activity, cut out body and head of an animal (a tree frog is in the Appendix), then cut additional rectangular pieces for legs and circles for eyes and toes. It's a good idea to trace the image onto paper so the child has an outline to work from.

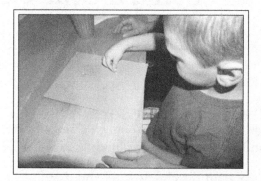

For a child fearful of touching school glue, do small projects such as putting toes on a tree frog. Be sure to keep a cup of water and a paper towel close by.

Scented, Colorful Dough

Here are two recipes for edible dough. One recipe has a gluten-free option. The first recipe optionally uses a fruit drink mix, and the second recipe calls for flavored gelatin. In both cases, use sugar-free products which will not mold as sugar does. You can find cream of tartar in the baking section of your grocery store.

Simple dough

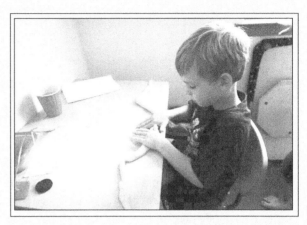

Boy making a snake using Jell-O dough.

- 1 cup of flour
- 1 cup of boiling water
- 2 tablespoons of cream of tartar
- 1/2 cup of salt
- 1 tablespoon of oil
- Optional: food dye and a drop of essential oil (for scent), or sugar-free Kool-Aid™ for color and scent.

Instructions: Mix these together with a large spoon, kneading the dough until firm. Form it into a ball and store it. It will keep for a month or more.

Safety hazard: Boiling water.

No-cook Jell-O™ dough

This dough has a pastel color and a silky texture. If you use sugar-free gelatin, it will store for a long time in the refrigerator.

- 1 3-ounce package of sugar-free gelatin
- 1 cup flour (can substitute all-purpose gluten free flour)
- 1 tablespoon cream of tartar or baking powder
- 1/4 cup salt
- 1 cup boiling water
- 2 tablespoons oil (avoid olive oil which will discolor it)
- Extra flour, as needed
- More flour to remove stickiness

Instructions:

1. Put the gelatin, flour, cream of tartar and salt in a bowl and whisk them together.
2. Add the boiling water and the oil.

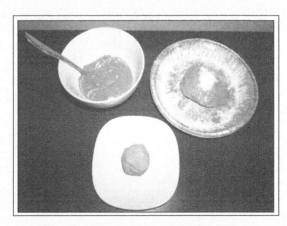

Top left: The bowl contains a very sticky dough mixture without the additional flour. Top right: Dough was transferred to a flat dish for kneading-in flour. Bottom: Some finished dough.

3. Stir with a spoon until the dough becomes unmanageable, and then knead it with your fingers, removing any lumps and mixing completely.

4. The dough will be sticky. Knead-in (add in) more flour. You might have to add quite a bit of flour to make the dough silky without a sticky texture.

5. Put it into a zip-lock bag in the refrigerator until you are ready for it. Return it to the refrigerator between uses to prolong its life.

Safety hazard: Boiling water.

Touch Activity 7

Cook's Helper

Once the child is able to face small amounts of messiness and messy fingers, being a cook's helper is an easy way to get additional exposure to new textures. Making a sandwich, stirring soup, making cookies, or peeling potatoes are easy ways to acclimate to the world of messy things. Your role is to give the child control over her task and let her do it in her own way and in her own time. We need to be patient as she develops the courage to face her fears and to learn new skills.

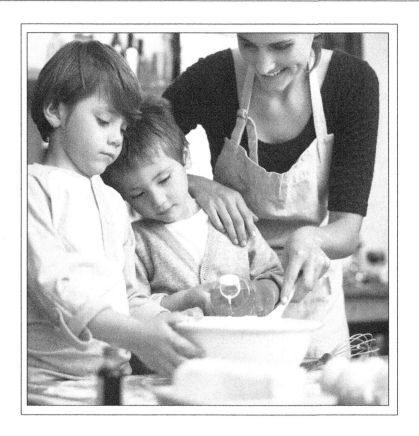

Birds Nest Cookies

Here is a delicious way to get children actively touching something gooey. These are no-bake cookies that are formed to look like bird nests. Put a few berries or jelly beans in them when they are chilled.

Materials: Microwave oven; bowl and spoon; measuring cups; baking sheet lined with waxed paper for shredded wheat version; paper cupcake liners and cupcake pan for coconut version.

Ingredients: Crunchy peanut butter (substitute nut butter or sunflower butter, if desired); chocolate chip bits (gluten-free, dairy free, soy free chips are available in health food stores); shredded wheat, All Bran™, or shredded coconut; berries or jelly beans. Use about 1 spoon each of cereal, chocolate chips and peanut butter for each nest.

1. Melt the chocolate chips in a glass or ceramic bowl in the microwave using moderate (level 5) power for about 1 minute. Use a mitt; the bowl will be very hot.
2. Place the cereal or coconut into a cup or bowl.
3. Add the chocolate and peanut butter and mix gently
4. Have the child take a heaping tablespoon of the mixture and shape it in to a nest. Place the nest on waxed paper or in a cupcake liner. Repeat until the batter is used.
5. Chill the nests. Optionally, add 2 or three berries for eggs.

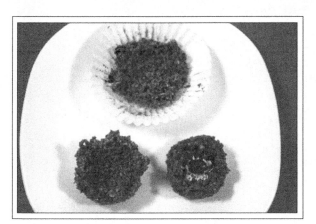

Birds nests

More

- See Taste Activity 3: *Food drawings and paintings.*
- See *Making bath bombs* in environmental enrichment, exercise 7.

Touch Immersion

Children (and adults) may find pleasure in various properties of objects (particularly natural objects). Glass, tile, stone and metal are smooth and cool to the touch. Fiber like yarn is soft and warm. Bread dough is gooey. Wood makes the transition from rough to smooth as we sandpaper it. Wood is cool to the touch, but less so than metal and glass. Seeds, beads and small stones can be manipulated between the fingers. Finger foods can be dry (bread, crackers), wet (peaches, melon), hot or cold, firm, mushy (bananas and French fries), oily, messy (bar-b-q chips) and so on.

Our brain senses these properties and may develop an attraction to them and sometimes a craving for them. The point of this section is to engage children in activities that appeal to them and calm them. You will want to explore the impact of the touch, temperature and manipulability characteristics on the children you work with so you can better understand which types of immersion activities will appeal to them.

Work with Yarn and Fibers

Here are a series of activities that are graded by skill starting with making pipe cleaner animals and simple yarn wrapping activities and ending with a multi-day project making a 20" yarn-doll monkey with cap. All of these tasks are within the skillset of a young child (in the case of the monkey doll, assistance is required from an adult for assembly of the pieces).

Goal: Calming through soft touch; to increase visual-motor skills.

Touch Activity 9

Pipe Cleaner Dolls

Materials: Pipe cleaners, both full size and a few cut and cut in half.

Instructions:

1. Roll one-half of a pipe cleaner into a ball for the head. Tuck the raw end into the ball.
2. Use a full length pipe cleaner to form the head, ears, body and tail.
3. Twist the ends tightly around the body and turn the raw ends into the fur.
4. Push the rolled ball into the shaped head and pinch it tight.
5. Use one-half of a pipe cleaner each for the front legs and the back legs. Center each set of legs in place over the body and twist them two or three times to secure them.
6. Bend the leg ends for feet and bend the tail.

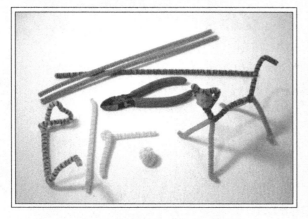

To make an animal, fashion a head, ears and tail from one pipe cleaner. Cut a second pipe cleaner in half to fashion the legs. Twist pieces tightly together and hide pointed ends.

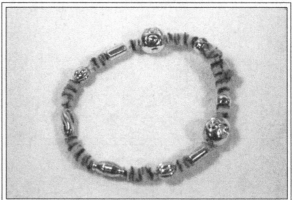

Make a simple beaded pipe cleaner bracelet. Be sure to hide the raw wire ends in the pipe cleaner fur.

104

Yarn Wrapping

Wrapping yarn is simple enough for a young child. The steady movement and soft yarn are calming.

Materials: Yarn; cardboard, paper tubes or jars; optional: glue, bowl of water and paper towel.

Instructions: Wrap yarn or string around cardboard, tissue tubes, or other cylindrical objects.

Decorate a tube, box or jar

Cover a section of the tube (box or jar) with school glue or a glue stick. Wrap lengths of different colored yarn around the tube. (Have a bowl of clean water and a towel nearby to rinse glue off fingers.)

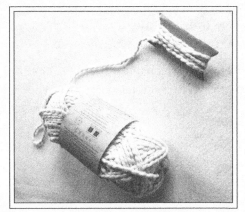

Yarn wrapping is easy enough for a small child to do. Children with touch sensitivity love the feel of soft yarn on their fingers.

Yarn Doll

Materials: Yarn; strips of cardboard or cardstock; string or more yarn for ties.

Instructions:

1. Wrap yarn around cardboard for the body.
2. Tie off the head with string.
3. At the opposite end, cut through the loops to make the legs.
4. Use a shorter piece of cardboard to wrap the arms.
5. Tie the ends of the arms with string and snip through the loops of yarn at each end.
6. Split the body in two parts (front and back, see photo.) Center the arms between them. Tie a string around the waist to secure the arms in place.
7. If making pant legs, split the yarn into two parts and tie each leg at the ankle with string. Leave untied for a skirt.

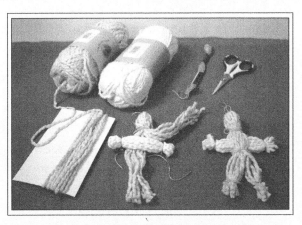

Make a yarn doll: Left side shows cardboard being wrapped with yarn. Right side shows the simple construction steps.

Touch Activity 12

Roll a Ball of Yarn

To wrap yarn into a ball: once past the first inch, lay each wrapping of yarn next to the previous wrapping while at the same time, turning the ball slightly. Wrap tightly, turning the ball in all directions as you wrap.

To prevent the ball from unwinding, put a small dab of school glue under several pieces of yarn while wrapping the final layer.

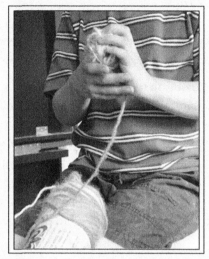

Boy rolling a ball of yarn.

Touch Activity 13

Yarn Chains

Instructions (reverse for left-handed child):

1. Unwrap about 2 feet (2/3 m.) of yarn from the ball.
2. At the yarn's end, make a knotted loop with a 2-3 inch (5 cm) tail.
3. Hold the tail firmly with the thumb and index finger of the left hand. Loosely hold the long end with the other fingers on the left hand.
4. Use the fingers of the right hand pull a small loop of yarn through the loop. Pull it tight. You now have a new loop.
5. If the new loop is too big, pull on the yarn to make it smaller—you want it large enough for your fingers to get through.
6. Continue making new loops until the chain is the length you want, then snip the yarn somewhere on the loop. Pull the end tight.

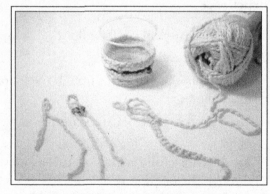

Materials for making yarn chains.

106

Yarn Chain Crafts

Decorate cups, boxes, jars and other objects with yarn chains by gluing the chains in circles around the cups. The chains can also be glued in spirals and squares to fit the object they are glued to. Consider using chains of complementary colors and consider adding beads to the yarn chains as you make them.

Combine all of the ideas for working with yarn together in one long project by creating the yarn monkey at the end of this chapter.

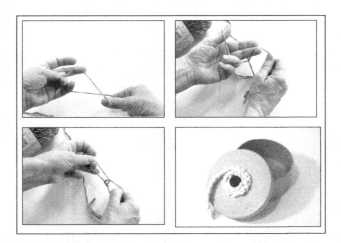

Left hand instructions for chaining are the reverse of right hand. Form a loop of the yarn, and then pull the long end through the loop, making a second loop. Hold the second loop and pull the long end tight. This is the first chain. The chain will grow as you continue making loops and pulling them tight. When you have a long enough chain, make one last loop and snip it at the top (of the loop). Pull the snipped end tight. Trim both ends of loose yarn, Bottom right: a portion of a yarn chain has been glued to small box lid.

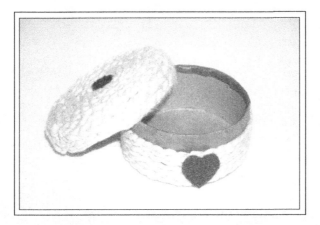

Finished box. The sides were covered with paper and then wrapped with yarn that was not chained. The heart is cut from felt.

Touch Activity 14

Project: Monkey Yarn Doll with Cap

Here is a multi-day project constructed of easy steps for the child with construction assistance from an adult. The monkey is made of yarn balls and wrapping. His hat is made of yarn chains glued to a plastic cup.

The instructions for this project can be found in chapter 11, Multiple-day projects.

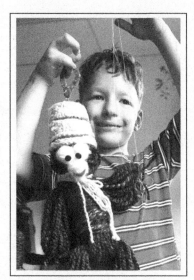

The finished monkey.

Glass, Stone, and Metal

Small children who like the cool touch of glass, metal, stone and tile will typically find themselves playing with things such as instruments and board games rather than creating things such as crafts. Older children might find pleasure in using wood-working tools for wood projects, making jewelry or in getting out the pots, pans, baking dishes and stirring spoons to cook and bake. Here are a few ideas for immersing children of all ages in the touch of cool, smooth objects.

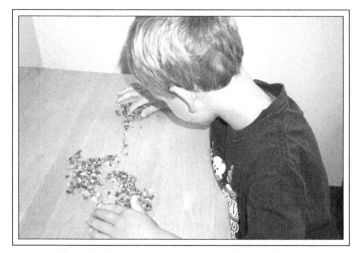

**Simply lining up stones can be soothing
for a child with autism.**

Stone Covered Jar or Cup

Stones are glued to the top of the cup. They must dry before the cup can be turned, so this activity requires 5-8 short sessions.

Materials: Pebbles, a plastic cup or glass jar, a container large enough to hold the cup; sand; school glue; a cup of water and a paper towel.

Instructions:

1. Put 1 inch (3 cm) of sand in the container. Put the cup into the container, scooping sand inside to weigh it down.
2. Put a thin coat of glue along the side of the cup that is facing up.
3. By hand, place pebbles on the glue.
4. Let it dry, turn the cup and repeat.

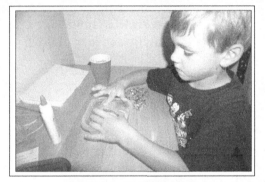

Boy is steadying a stone he has placed on the cup.

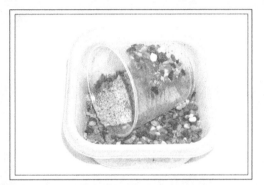

Sand inside the cup holds it in place. Glue stones to the top and let dry.

Tile Mosaic with Glass Stones or Pebbles

Materials: Different colored glass stones; a used cd disc, an old plate or square of corrugated cardboard, school glue; a cup of water and a paper towel.

Instructions:

1. Make an interesting design or picture using the stones or pebbles.
2. Transfer the stones to the CD or plate and glue them in place.

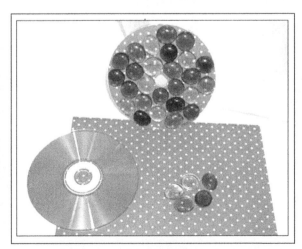

A used CD is covered first with paper and then with glass beads.

Metal Pen and Pencil and Drawing Tools

Metal or mechanical pencils are uncommon today, but metal pens can still be found as give-aways from merchants and as the higher-price option in an office supply store. These are the ultimate touch fidget for a child who rubs his fingers on objects. In addition, metal (aluminum) drawing and drafting tools such as rulers, angles, compasses and protractors can be found at reasonable prices at art and drafting supply stores and websites.

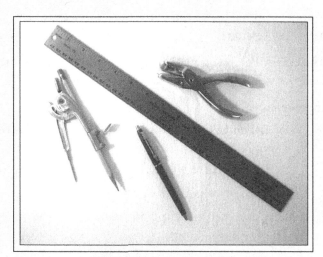

**Metal drawing tools for
the analytic sensory child.**

Start a Coin Collection

Collecting coins can provide a child with hours of tactile and visual fun. There is an added thrill in finding a 1949 penny in mom's pocket change. Get a spare folder to hold unusual or old coins.

Materials: Pennies or quarters; inexpensive coin folders (found online or in some coin shops.)

Instructions: Sort coins into the folders. When there are doubles, keep the best coin.

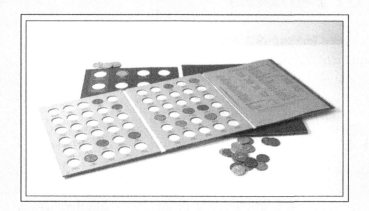

Touch Activity 19

Musical Instruments

Playing an instrument is an excellent way to get touch immersion. And using an instrument for touch immersion is an excellent way to learn to play, since one must "practice, practice, practice." Here are some instruments that produce the cool touch response. See the section on sound for more about musical instruments.

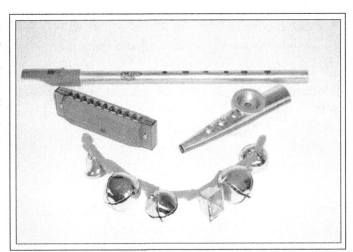

Metal instruments that are smooth and cool to the touch can satisfy a touch craving in some children.

- Stringed instruments with metal strings or parts (guitars, electric bass, dulcimer and so on)
- Horns and whistles
- Percussion such as spoons, cowbells and triangles

Touch Activity 20

Games with Tile, Stone or Metal Pieces

Many games have interesting textures. Look for used versions with stone tiles or pieces.

- Dominos
- Checkers
- Chess
- Go
- Mahjong
- Erector sets

Wood

The rich sensation of smoothly sanded wood appeals to some children. The activities presented here provide a good introduction to woodwork for children five years and older. Younger children may enjoy playing with unfinished wooden toys, Tinker Toys™ and Jenga™.

Sanding Wood

A child enamored with the feel of wood will enjoy the silky feeling of the sanded object and the texture of the wood grain.

Materials: A small piece of pine or other soft wood with an interesting grain pattern; sandpaper: 100, 150 and 220 grit; a tack cloth; optional: a small unfinished wood object such as a birdhouse or car (available at craft shops).

Instructions: Sand the wood first with the rougher (100 and 150 grit) sandpaper. Wipe it clean with tack cloth; Repeat with the 220 grit sandpaper.

Safety hazard: Avoid exotic woods, redwood, red cedar and western cedar which can be allergenic. Pine is a safe choice.

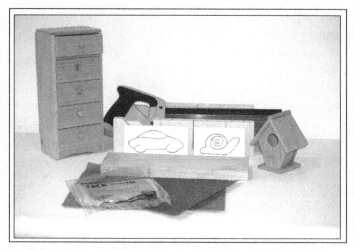

Here are several different sanding activities: a tiny set of drawers or a birdhouse (both from craft stores), or cut out a snail or car with adult cutting tools.

Sanding Wooden Objects

Cut a shape for a child to sand. The car and snail illustrations in the Appendix can be cut from a 1 x 4-inch board.

Materials: A piece of 1 x 4-inch pine board; sandpaper: 100, 150 and 220 grit; a tack cloth; tools: a jigsaw or coping saw; car and snail illustrations in the Appendix.

Instructions:

1. Draw the image onto the board.
2. Use a coping saw or a jigsaw to cut out the object.
3. Have the child sand the wood first with the rougher (100 and 150 grit) sandpaper. Wipe it clean with tack cloth. Repeat with the 220 grit sandpaper.
4. Optionally, add the details from the drawing of the snail or car using a pen or a knife (older child under supervision).

Touch Activity 23

Building A Truck

This activity involves simple sawing and drilling that is easy enough for an older child (or a non-handy adult) to perform.

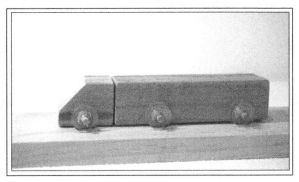

Making a truck is only a bit more work than making a car.

Materials: 2 x 2 inch pine wood; 6 sewing machine bobbins for wheels (found at fabric shops); dowel rod to fit inside bobbins; sandpaper; a tack cloth; tools: a miter box and saw or a wood saw; a drill, glue.

Instructions:

1. Cut a 5 inch (12 cm) piece of wood for the trailer.
2. Cut a 2 inch (5 cm) piece of wood for the cab and cut off a corner to make the windshield.
3. Drill holes above the bottom edge for the axel (dowel rod) to fit through (see photo).
4. Cut three lengths of dowel rod to equal the car's width plus the width of two wheels.
5. Thread each dowel rod through the car body and wheels, glue it to both wheels. (The wheels will turn on the axels.)
6. Attach the cab to the trailer with glue or a fastener.

Safety hazard: Avoid exotic woods, redwood, red cedar and western cedar which can be allergenic. Pine is a safe choice.

Touch Activity 24

Gooey Revisited

Doughs and clays are useful both for sensory immersion and for touch desensitization. Many dough products are available on the market, as well as many recipes for making dough (see the above section of tactile desensitization).

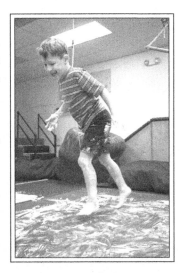

For some children, acclimation to gooey substances is no problem. In fact, they might prefer messy things. Along with standard activities like finger painting, working with clay, playing with slime toys and playing in mud, here are additional ideas for the older child who seeks gooey sensation.

- Baking cookies
- Kneading bread or pizza dough
- Gardening
- Papier mache
- Paper making

Taste and Smell

Desensitization to the Sensation of Food

Playing with food is a good way to help desensitize a child to the touch, smell, sight and taste of different foods. Food play is not done at mealtime, when the goal is to ingest the food, but at another time of the day when the intention is to gain tolerance to foods. As an exercise for a very picky eater, it should be done frequently. Here is an example of using play with a child who is a picky eater.

Place bits of food in front of the child and let him play with them. Show him how to make a house out of cubes of cheese and draw stick figures with spaghetti or pieces of rice. Use ketchup and ranch dressing as finger paints. In this way, the child slowly gets used to the color, smell, texture and sizes of a variety of foods. He can feel the food's crunchiness or mushiness. He can squeeze it, press it or pull it apart. When the child has gotten used to handling food, he is ready for any number of interesting activities. He could help his parents prepare meals by washing vegetables, or opening cans or scooping food out of the jar into a bowl. He can carry food from the stove to the table. All of this continues the desensitization process. We still have not yet asked him to eat the food, but we'll do so slowly with just a drop or just a lick. We might add a small amount of the new food to foods he already likes. With time, we continue to gently increase his exposure to a variety of new foods.

Food desensitization can be a lengthy process. In some situations, we can speed up the process by increasing the number of exposures in a day to new foods.

Consider the challenge of desensitizing a child to the smell of eggs. You could put some cooked eggs into a jar and reward the child when she opens the lid and takes a quick sniff. You can make a game of this in which she tries to keep the jar open for longer periods of time while keeping a straight face. Eventually she will become accustomed to the smell of the eggs.

Who is doing this desensitization? It could be a parent, clinician, teacher or therapist at school. If you are doing this in the clinic or at school, try to involve the parent in the intervention so that it more readily transfers to home. Transitioning feeding gains to the home setting is the most difficult step of the desensitization process.

In many households, parents try to limit exposure to sugars, food coloring, and crunchy snacks with salt and fat. While this is an admirable goal, we sometimes break the rules (all the rules!) when working with the very picky eater. We can find a "way in" to the picky eater's difficulties by making food sweeter, saltier, or more colorful. But once the child is eating these new foods, we will need to slowly decrease the level of the tempters (salt, sugar, fat, coloring) we have deployed. Meanwhile, it is a good idea to avoid artificial ingredients. Two-to-three percent of children become hyperactive when given food coloring (especially the reds and yellows) and some food additives, notably sodium benzoate found in sodas.

Safety Considerations: Food sensitivities and allergies are common in children with autism and not uncommon in children with other neurodevelopmental disorders such as ADHD and sensory processing disorders. Always ask parents about known or suspected food issues. If a child has never eaten a particular food that is a known allergen (such as soy or tree nuts), proceed slowly and keep an eye out for rashes, behaviors and bowel changes.

These activities from other chapters also have taste or smell input:

Touch activity, Ch. 6	Vision, Ch. 9
#6, Scented dough	#13, Collage with dried flowers and leaves
#7, Cook's helper	
#8, Birds' nests	

Food Activity 1

Gelatin Shapes

Make a sheet of gelatin and then cut it into play shapes.

Materials: One packet of gelatin; water or juice; bowl; cookie cutters or knife; spatula; Optional: bits of fruit for decoration. Unflavored, uncolored gelatin is available in grocery stores. Use grape, orange or apple juice to flavor it.

1. Heat ¾ cup of water and bring to a boil.
2. In a bowl, sprinkle the gelatin powder on top of the cold water or juice. Let it sit for one minute.
3. Add the hot water or juice and stir until it is completely dissolved.
4. Pour into a baking dish and refrigerate until it is firm to the touch.

Have the child use cookie cutters or a butter knife to cut the gelatin into shapes. Remove the shapes with a spatula. Create pictures, stack the blocks, or decorate them with bits of fruit.

Food Activity 2

Dolphins and Starfish for Breakfast

This is a novel way to increase a child's interest in eating breakfast. For the very picky eater, introduce these foods during a play session where the goal is to explore rather than eat.

Materials: Regular or gluten-free, dairy-free bread; egg; apple. For decoration: peanut butter, nut butter or apple butter; jam; berries. Fish shaped cookie cutters or a knife and the fish patterns in Appendix of this book (trace the shapes onto waxed paper).

1. Dolphin scrambled egg:
   a. Scramble an egg in a bowl and gently cook it in a pan. Turn it over when it is no longer runny. Cook gently on the other side and remove before it is brown.
   b. Use cookie cutters to cut shapes of the egg, or use a knife and the pattern in this book to cut two dolphin shapes.
2. Fish toast:
   a. Toast a slice of bread. Cut fish shapes in the toast. Decorate it with peanut butter or apple butter, jam and berries.
3. Sand dollar apple
   a. Peel an apple, then cut horizontal slices. Use the star shape center of the apple as your guide to cutting out a star (the core) from the slice.

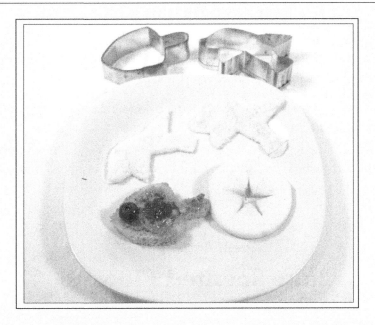

Dolphin eggs, fish toast with a blueberry eye and a starfish apple. Here is food that can be played with before it goes "down the hatch!"

Food Activity 3

Food Drawings and Paintings

Children can use all kinds of foods to make pictures during a play session. Here is a follow-up activity to the "food man" drawing in environmental enrichment exercise one. In this activity, the goal is exploration of foods. Once the child is comfortable with a given color, texture and smell, you might suggest that she put a dab on her tongue. Have a preferred food nearby to taste afterward as both a palate cleanser and a reward.

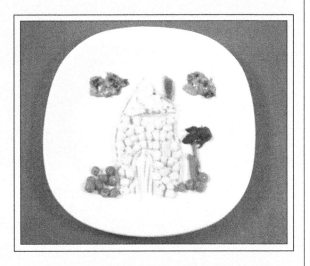

Spaghetti outlines the house, and forms the door and window. Corn is used for siding; the roof is corn chips; the chimney is catsup; the grass is peas and broccoli is used for the tree. Blueberries mashed into yogurt were used to paint clouds.

- Use frozen, canned or fresh vegetables to draw pictures of flowers, houses, robots and so on.

- Use catsup, mustard and ranch and French dressings for finger paints. Mashed blueberries, carrots, peas or broccoli can provide additional colors. Add colorful juice (carrot, grape or cherry) to yogurt or salad dressing to make pastel colors.

- Cooked spaghetti can be used to make the lines of objects like animals and houses.

- Look through your cupboards for soy sauce, molasses, jams, honey, tomato paste and other food items than can be useful during playtime.

Scent Immersion

Scent is craved by some children and found to be invasive to others. The treatment of scent immersion in this chapter utilizes a small amount of scent and places access to the scent under the child's control. For additional information see "Using scents" in chapter 3. Also, follow these cautions:

- When using new scents or exposing the child to fragrant flowers, keep an eye out for signs of allergic reaction such as sneezing, rashes, stuffy nose, or scratchy throat.
- When using scents with children, stick to kitchen herbs and spices and known flowers. Herbs typically used in adult aromatherapy, such as lavender and eucalyptus, are not necessarily suitable for children.
- Do not sniff loose spices. They can irritate nasal passages.

Scent Activity 1

Make Scented Flowers

Here is a delightful way to provide a child with scent. The centers of the flowers are made of a natural fabric such as cotton or wool that will hold the scent of essential oil for a day or two. Add additional scent when needed.

Materials: Felt squares in different colors; scraps of natural fabric (cotton, linen, silk, wool hemp or bamboo); stapler; school glue; needle and thread or epoxy; several different bottles of fruit or flower scented essential oil; flower petal and center patterns (found in the Appendix).

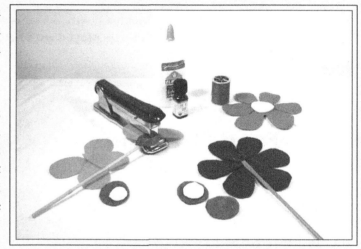

Left flower petals are being stapled to center. Bottom: Straw has been stapled to the back side and the flower is ready for cotton and finish felt centers. Top right flower is complete.

1. Cut out six petals and two centers (circles) of felt for each flower.
2. Cut out one center (circle) of cotton. Trim it so that it is a little smaller than the felt circles. Set it aside.
3. Arrange petals around one of the centers and staple them. The staple prongs should be on the back (petal) side.
4. Flatten one end of a straw and staple it to the back side. The prong end is on the petal side.
5. Glue together the remaining felt center and the cotton center with school glue, and then glue that to the backside of the flower.
6. To make the flower secure, put a stitch or two through all the centers. Or have an adult put small dabs of permanent glue on the edges of the centers. Leave the middle of the center free of permanent glue—this is where the scent goes.
7. Add a drop of essential oil to the center. It will scent the cotton for a day or two.

Safety hazard: be aware of allergies when choosing the essential oil scents.

Make Medallion Necklace

1. **Materials:** Small pieces of felt; small pieces of cotton, linen, wool or silk; leather or cotton or a novelty band for a "necklace;" hole punch, glue, scissors, essential oil.

Medallion

a. Cut two identical shapes from felt. Optionally, use white felt and decorate it with ink, marker or paint.

b. Cut a piece of natural fabric (cotton, linen, wool) smaller than the first shape.

c. Arrange the pieces in order: felt, cotton, felt. Use a hole-punch or scissors to make a small hole through all three pieces. If they are too thick, mark each and punch them one at a time.

d. Glue the felt shapes together at the edges, avoiding the area with the cotton fabric. The scent will go there.

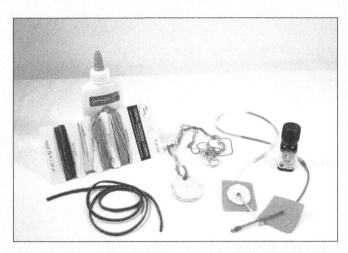

Make the scented medallion cover from fabric such as felt. Use natural fabric inside the cover to wick the scent. Leather, cotton chain or novel materials can be used for the necklace.

Band

a. Purchase a fashionable band, ribbon, or cord. Cut it to size.

b. Optionally, make a cord chain (see Touch activity 13). Leave long strings at each end for ties.

2. Put the band or cord through the hole in the medallion and fasten the ends.

3. Each day, place a drop of essential oil at the center of the medallion.

Make Teas to Drink or Scent the Room

Teas have a wonderful fragrance that can calm the senses as you drink them. The teas listed in the materials list are non-caffeinated and are appropriate for children. Avoid unusual and medicinal herbs including lavender which may cause side-effects for children.

Materials: Dried herbs such as cinnamon, fennel seeds, chamomile, rosebuds, sage, lemon balm, citrus rind, and hibiscus. These are often available in bulk in health stores and online.

- Brew one tablespoon of herbs in a cup of boiling water for 5-10 minutes.
- Boil spices like cinnamon in a pot for 10-15 minutes. For a strong but pleasant fragrance, try cooking cinnamon and rosebuds together.
- To add fragrance to a room, put herbs or spices in a pot and let simmer for 15-20 minutes.

Grow Your Own Plants

Consider growing pots of the herbs at home or school so that fresh herbs are on hand or shop at the bulk bins for dried orange and lemon rind, dried roses and spices

Grow indoor or outdoor plants:

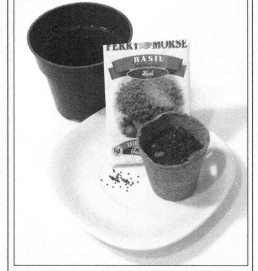

1. Herb garden: Two kid-friendly herbs are mint and lemon balm

2. Kitchen garden: Other fragrant herbs that are easily grown indoors are basil, chives, thyme, sage, rosemary, oregano, tarragon, cardamom and parsley

3. Fragrant flowers: Rose, lilac, lily of the valley, gardenia and others – but watch for allergies

4. African violets (for visual stimulation rather than for scent)

5. Small pine or bonsai in the home

Materials: small peat pots; potting soil; seeds; permanent pots.

1. Put potting soil into peat pots. Optionally, you can plant the peat pot in a second bigger pot to help it retain moisture.

2. Put two seeds into a pot together and cover them with 1/4-1/2 inch (.5 cm – 1 cm) of soil (see recommended coverage on the seed package). Tamp down the soil.

3. Water the seeds.

4. Put the plant in a sunny location: outside (in warm weather), or on a sunny window sill or under a grow light. Keep the soil moist. In hot environments, water the seeds often and protect the pot from too much sun. When the plant is 2-3 inches tall, transfer the peat pot with plant into its permanent dish.

Pocketful of Scent for a Child

Here's a way to give a child natural scent each day. Use fresh herbs and a bit of flower (whatever is blooming indoors or outdoors) to make a small corsage or boutonniere. Or put a sprig of mint or lemon balm in his pocket. He can get the scent on his fingers by rubbing the herb through the day.

If fresh herbs are out of the question, then try ½ teaspoon of dry herbs in small sachet, pill container or simply in the pocket. To keep the scent strong, replace the herbs every 1-2 days.

More Ideas for Scent

1. Do crafts such as collages and mosaics using flower petals, herbs and seeds and citrus rind for the materials.
2. Make scented lotions. (See section on scent in the materials section of the environmental enrichment protocol.)
3. Burn incense at home (under adult supervision).

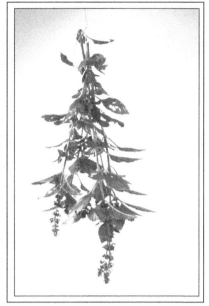

Grow herbs and fragrant flowers in pots or a garden. Harvest them (clip them) and hang them upside down in a cool, dry place to dry. When they are dry enough to crumble, store them in jars for scents in the winter.

Multi-Sensory Dish Garden

Make a planter, then fill it with plants and décor. This is a multi-day project with many different sensory components: the earthy smell of the soil, desensitization to touch and immersion in touch as the child coats a dish in sand and pebbles; visual immersion through sorting colored pebbles and making a pattern with them; and the sensory aspects of the plants themselves.

The instructions for this project can be found in chapter 11, Multiple-day projects.

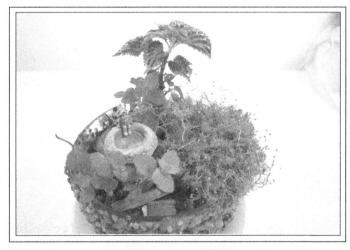

Planter contains mint (scent) moss (touch) and coleus (visual). They were planted in potting soil and have a woodchip covering. Pebbles would work, too.

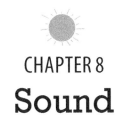

CHAPTER 8

Sound

Sound can make us tear up with its beauty and alarm us with its might. As with the other senses, children can crave it, avoid it or be oblivious to its presence in the environment. This chapter contains strategies and activities to help desensitize a child to sound as well as fun activities to immerse a child in it.

Sound Desensitization

Sound sensitivity is a hearing system dysfunction in which normal sounds and sound volumes are magnified and can cause discomfort. A child with sound sensitivity may develop an aversion to certain sounds, noises and voice registrations of normal volume, as well as to loud sounds. The observable symptoms of sound sensitivity vary. Some children wince with discomfort, others block their ears and still others act out with negative behaviors. Some can associate noises with discomfort and automate a negative response, through various learned behaviors.

Sound sensitivity is not currently repairable, and we do not currently have hearing products to decrease sensitive hearing other than blocking the ears with ear plugs or ear muffs. However, hearing aid technology has made great gains and perhaps in the near future there will be hearing devices that reduce the sounds that enter the ear.

Other problems such as temporary ear infections and tinnitus can also cause pain and an adverse reaction to certain sounds. Ear infections can be medically treated. However, there is little treatment for tinnitus other than to teach the child to relax and not focus on the offending sounds.

Before presenting the sound desensitization activities, we revisit some sound desensitization strategies from my previous book, *Self-Regulation Interventions and Strategies*:

- Decrease the noise in the child's environments so that her auditory processing, fear centers and emotional systems are not working so hard. Place rugs and mats on the floor and pictures and wall coverings on the walls to dampen sound. In a classroom setting, consider installing sound reduction tiles on classroom walls to help dampen sound. A preliminary study showed some effect (Kinnealy, 2012).

- Let the child use ear plugs and ear muffs in noisy environments like the school cafeteria.

- Give the child an alternate setting for situations that are too difficult (the cafeteria, music or gym class, and so on).

- Solve specific sound problems. For example, try to block noise outside the environment with calm music, or use a white noise machine to cover the sounds.

- Train the ear to accept particularly difficult sounds by recording the sounds and playing them back at a reduced volume throughout the day – with the child in control of the volume. (This technique comes from Temple Grandin.)

De-Coupling Sound Sensitivity and Learned Behaviors

There are times when a child with sound sensitivities gets "stuck" on certain sounds or noises (his sister chewing with her mouth open, his neighbor's dog barking, or a classmate giggling). The sound has bothered him in the past and he has developed a hair-trigger response when he hears it. When he hears those sounds, he might react with anger and tell the perpetrator to "shut up." Another child would tune out those sounds, but this child's brain is on the alert for them and ready with an inappropriate response.

An adult with these issues could break through them by practicing a combination of mindfulness and *loving kindness*, a technique that teaches empathy and compassion. Here is a scaled down version of those practices to help children with sensitivities combat both the feeling of irritation and the learned reaction of rage. Our example works with the sound of a child's sister chewing with her mouth open.

Materials: Sound recorder such as the voice memo function of a cell phone or tablet; paper; colored pens or pencils.

Instructions: This activity is performed over several sessions. Try to do it daily for a week, and then continue as needed thereafter. You can elect to work with one issue (e.g. the sound of chewing) or with multiple sounds and situations within a single setting.

1. Record the child's sister chewing with her mouth open. Set it aside.
2. Sessions 1-3:
   a. In a quiet room, have the child sit with his eyes looking downward (lightly closed) and feel the sensation of his breath as it moves in and out. Do this for seven minutes, occasionally reminding him to pay attention to his breath.
   b. Put out the paper and pens and ask the child to list three good things about his sister. Next, list three things that she struggles with such as breathing with her mouth closed, learning her spelling words, or making friends. Finally, list three nice things she has done for him.
   c. Draw a picture of his sister looking happy, doing something nice for him or doing something she enjoys.
   d. Write a sentence wishing for something good to happen to her, such as, "I hope you always have a lot of friends."
3. Session 4:
   a. Perform a shortened version of step two: watch the breathing for five minutes, list three good things about his sister, and then imagine her looking happy.
   b. Tell him that he will be attending to his breath again, but this time, you will occasionally play a recording of his sister's chewing with the volume turned low.
   c. Have him sit mindfully again for five minutes.
      i. After 30 seconds of his quiet breathing, tell him to wish for something nice for his sister and then to return to quiet breathing.

ii. Play the recording for 10 seconds, first telling him that if he feels anger, just replace it with a kind wish for his sister.

iii. Repeat this 10-second exercise two or three more times.

4. During subsequent sessions, increase the duration and the volume of the sound until it reaches its original volume.

Sound Activity 2
Listening Therapy with Bone Conduction

Listening therapy is a long-term program in which children (and adults) listen to specially enhanced music. The goal is to help reduce behaviors due to sound sensitivity. While there are no large studies that show the effectiveness of these products, there are thousands of individual case studies written by therapists showing that they help reduce unwanted behaviors. It appears that the technology works for some children and not others. Unfortunately, we do not yet know how to screen for children who would benefit from this type of program. A good strategy is to do a trial program for a few weeks prior to the family investing in the cost of the equipment.

Listening programs come both with and without a feature called bone conduction. Bone conduction, which provides sounds through vibration (on the skull) as well as sounds through headphones is thought to be a stronger treatment. There are several products on the market: Therapeutic Listening, The Listening Program; iLs (Integrated Listening Systems); and Samonas. Additional programs such as Berard Auditory Integration Training are offered by developmental audiologists. Most programs require 30-60 minutes per day of passive listening to classical music for a period of two or more months.

Sound Immersion

The activities presented in this section on sound immersion cover two distinct sets of needs. First are activities for children who get pleasure from music, sound rhythms and singing. This might be a child with sound sensitivities, or a child who craves sound.

Second are activities for children who struggle to make sense of what they hear. This may be a child with autism, or a child with poor sound sensitivity, or a child who has difficulty processing sounds. For the most part, the activities described here are useful for both sets of situations.

We can immerse children with autism in words, rhymes, picture books and non-verbal gestures as a way of introducing vocabulary, usage and sentence structure. The non-verbal child will make use of the activities below to gain reading and writing skills and, perhaps one day, speaking skills. He can utilize simple words and gestures to express his needs, wants and desires and to be heard. These activities give him a sense of control, without which he might become powerless or take control through act-out behaviors.

Reading Aloud

Children develop vocabulary and learn about the world through reading books and being read to by caregivers. Reading aloud is one of the most important activities parents and educators can do with a young child. A list of books for children with delayed speech and autism is in the Appendix.

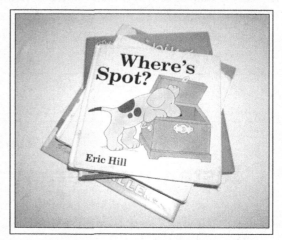

Develop vocabulary

Some books are better than others for developing vocabulary—both nouns, verbs, phrasing, as well as for the acquisition of facts. Picture books of objects such as animals and fruit can help to build the initial vocabulary a child with autism needs.

Developing thinking skills

Stories that ask questions on one page ("Is that a walrus?") and give the answer on the next ("No, it's an elephant!") provide an opportunity for the child to think and reply.

Teaching verbs

Verbs are harder to learn than nouns. They are less concrete and there are tenses to learn—past, present and future, as well as conjugations. Learning verbs and how to use them correctly is cumbersome for any child—and much more so for children with special needs. Here are two activities to help the struggling child:

Using gestures: We can teach children simple verbs with the aid of gestures. Here are straightforward examples.

- Walk – two fingers "walking" on a table.
- Run – fingers "walk" faster.
- Eat – bring an imaginary fork to mouth.

Reading books: Reading books can, with time, imprint verb endings into the child's mind. Two books that help with early verbs are Richard Lederer's, "I Can Play That" and Joy Cowley's, "Meanies." Reading lots of books out loud to the child and asking simple (or complicated) questions are the best ways to develop phrases with verbs.

Develop verbal rhythm

Phrases that repeat within the story help the child practice word groups. Word rhythm and rhyme help with vocabulary and phrase memorization, and can add to humor. Two popular examples of books with rhyming, repetitive phrases are Audrey Wood's, *The Napping Book* and *Green Eggs and Ham* by Dr. Seuss.

Here is a familiar example of rhyming, repetitive phrases from the 1700s.

As I was walking to St. Ives
I met a man with seven wives.
Each wife had seven sacks.
Each sack had seven cats.
Each cat had seven kits.
Kits, cats, sacks, wives, how many were going to St. Ives?

(You will remember that the answer is one. Just "I" am going to St. Ives; the man and his wives were not going anywhere.)

Sound Activity 4

Gestures

Learning gestures and signs can be an important step in developing verbal language skills in children with autism and other special needs. Studies show that communication skills are significantly improved when parents incorporate gestures into their verbal communication. Both formal signing such as ASL (American Sign Language) and informal made-up gestures work.

Using gestures

Make every sentence an opportunity to combine speech and gestures when talking to a non-verbal child.

What was said: *"C'mon, Rajiv! Let's walk to the playground."*

Gestures for each verb:

1. The beckoning arm swing for "come;"
2. Walking fingers for walk;
3. Arms moving as if to climb a ladder, or a hand that imitates sliding by first moving up and then "whooshing" down, accompanied by a verbal "whoosh."

Record Sound Effects

Recording sounds using an electronic device is a fun way for a child to spend hours of time. Use this activity with a child who craves noise and sound, as well as with a child who doesn't attend to sound.

Materials: A phone, tablet or music device with a voice recording app. You want one that can save the sounds by whatever name you provide.

Instructions:

1. Record a sound and save it.
2. Play it back and check that it is good.
3. Name the sound on your device so that you can find it again.

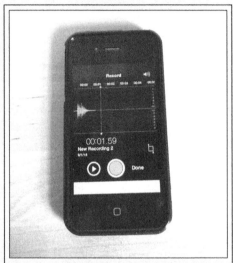

Use the Voice Memo or Audio Notes app on a cellphone to record sound effects. Name them so that you quickly find them to use in a story.

Below are some fun sounds to record. Also record fake sound effects with your mouth (screeching tires, whistling wind, a baby crying, and so on). You can use the sounds later as the sound effects for stories (see the activity below).

a. Closing a door

b. Opening the fridge

c. Running water

d. Saying your name

e. Walking noisily

f. Snapping fingers

g. "Hi {your name}"

h. Chewing crunchy food (apple, celery, carrot, chips) with mouth open

i. Chewing crunchy food with mouth closed (place microphone near mouth)

j. TV in the background

k. Music in the background

l. Doorbell

m. Knocking on the door

n. Clapping hands (like applause)

o. Buzzing like a bee

p. Mouth noises

q. Sounds at the dinner table

r. Traffic in the background

s. Pouring milk, water, or soda into a glass

t. Yelling: "Get up, (your name)!"

u. "Oh-h, no-o"

Make a Story with Sound Effects

Use the sound effects from the previous activity as part of a story. Here is a sample story to get you started.

Materials: Recorded sound effects from previous activity.

Instructions:

1. Write a story that includes sound effects. (Start with the one below.)
2. Read the story and play back the recorded sounds to make the sound effects.

My Morning

I was sound asleep [snore] when my brother walked into the room [walking] and yelled, "Get up, [your name]."

I woke up [yawning] and got out of bed [creaking].

I took a shower [water], brushed my teeth and used mouth wash [gurgle].

Mom had cereal on the table. I poured milk in the bowl [splash], then ate crunchy cereal [CHOMP-CHOMP].

"Hey don't chew so loud!" my brother said. "Okay," I replied. I closed my mouth and chewed. [chomp-chomp].

I rinsed my bowl [splashing] and set it down [clink].

Julian came over. ["Hey, Joe!"]

We went outside [creaking, slamming] and played our favorite game: who can make the silliest rhyme ("slime!!!").

Julian said, "Ogre, booger."

"That doesn't rhyme," I said. "Let me try. Rest, pest."

"Rest, pest!" Julian said. "That's lame. Here's one, 'wiper' 'diaper'."

"You win!"

The Silliest Rhyme

Here's a fun game for children who love to talk. This can be played with two or more children.

Materials: Optional: a children's dictionary as an aid in thinking of words.

Instructions:

1. Each child is asked to think up a silly rhyme. You can preselect the words or have the children think them up. Vote on which is silliest. Here is a starter set: Crow, tree, dog, tub, fun, brick, and page.
2. Have the children make sentences or two-sentence poems with their silly words.

Make Silly Songs

Add rhythms to rhymes in this fun game.

1. Think of rhyming words: pie, sky, spy, cry, eye, why, sigh.

2. Create some silly sentences:

The pie fell from the sky.

It hit the spy in the eye.

3. Put rhythm to the rhyming words and keep going until you have a silly poem.

> The apple pie fell out of the sky,
> It hit the spy right in the eye.
> Said the spy, "Please tell me why
> An apple pie could land in my eye."
> I heard him sigh, I heard him cry,
> But no one ever told him why.
> Why not lemon, why not rye?
> Why a falling apple pie?
> You think I joke, you think I lie.
> But don't look up! Don't even try!
> I tell you, don't look in the sky!
> A falling pie might land in your eye.

4. Sing it to a simple tune.

Music

Nothing can compete with music as an immersion activity. Immerse a child in the types of music he likes, and teach him, through exposure, to like new types of music. Immerse him in singing, dancing and listening. And consider teaching him an instrument.

Sound Activity 9

Make or Obtain Simple Instruments

Make or find simple instruments to play while singing or listening to favorite tunes.

1. Homemade drums and sticks
2. Kazoo, comb and waxed paper, spoons
3. Chimes, gongs, bells

Also, clap and stamp to the beat of music.

To make a program:

1. Set up a daily or weekly schedule
2. Plan activities
3. Plan how you will increase the challenge
4. Stick to the plan

CHAPTER 9

Visual Immersion

With the abundance of visual electronic stimulation in our lives, you might think that children hardly need additional visual input. However, in spite of all that stimulation, a child might be missing the *right* type of input. The goal of sensory immersion is to provide the child with pleasure and satisfaction in choosing just the right elements for a functional item for school or a bit of decoration for her room. We want her to immerse herself in visual sensation that comforts and energizes her. This chapter contains many activities to do just that.

The elements of visual stimulation include the interplay of multiple colors, movement, lines, shapes, patterns, and the level of detail. One child might be drawn to intricate paisleys, another to bright or contrasting colors and chaotic dots, and yet another child might prefer soothing colors or orderly patterns of lines or checks. Each child's need for stimulating or calming sensation will change from day-to-day and vary with the time of day and the season.

Soft colors, detailed lines and complementary patterns such as calico take us inward. These elements help support and calm the child dealing with the angst of sensory overload. Colors and forms from nature have soft colors and lines that are soothing to look at.

Bright colors and simple lines support overt emotions like joy, anger and excitement. Man-made designs such as mazes, plaids and angular designs are alerting and organize the brain. If a child is rigid, linear patterns may appeal to him on a regular basis. When he is upset, rounder, softer lines may be soothing.

Along with colored pens, pencils, paints, markers and glue, the types of materials useful for visual projects for children include scrapbooking paper, gift-wrap paper, scraps of fabric with texture, interesting prints like calico, plain fabric (for borders and contrast), ribbons, and scrap sewing bindings. Old wallpaper and upholstery sample books are a good source for paper and fabric with interesting color and texture combinations. Consider keeping on hand a selection of decorative materials such as glitters, stones, bits of wood, glass stones, and dried leaves and flowers. Useful tools for visual projects are scissors, glues, a paper cutter or a shredder (for making ribbons of paper), and pinking shears for fabric.

Present the child with a choice of materials and colors. Discover her color and pattern preferences by paging through books on patterns and designs (from a library or online). Try to determine what she is drawn to when she is sad versus when she is having a good day.

On a typical day you may want to give him activities involving lines, letters and numbers. But on a day where he is sullen or overwhelmed, consider making use of natural materials and softer shapes. Some children are enchanted by glittering objects, so glitter, glass stones or mirrors can add to a project's appeal.

Consider setting up a visual immersion project to run across multiple days and to give the child a visual break. Several such projects are included in this chapter.

These activities from earlier chapters are also good for visual immersion:

Touch activity, Ch. 6	Food activity, Ch. 7	Scent activity, Ch. 7	Sound activity, Ch. 8
#3, Bunny picture	#3, Drawing with food	#6, Planter	#2, Reading books
#4, Simple collage			
#5, Frog picture			
#14, Gluing pebbles			
#17, Metal drawing tools			
#18, Sorting coins			

Coloring, Drawing & Puzzles

Children are naturally drawn to visual art activities. Use a 10-15-minute break during the day to immerse the child in visual sensations.

Materials: Paper; pencils; crayons, water paints, colored markers or pencils; coloring books.

Let's color something

It's easy to find pages for small children to color. For an older child, use pages from an adult coloring book or one of the many design books on the market that feature paisley, ethnic or nature designs, or stained glass windows.

Let's draw something

Give the child paper, a pencil and coloring materials. Suggest a picture to draw. There are several suggestions below. Keep the focus on having fun. It is important not to judge the results.

1. Draw me a picture of your day.
2. What would you do if you could do anything? Draw a picture of it.
3. Think of a day in which you received a big, happy surprise. Draw a picture of it.
4. Draw the view from your window.
5. Draw your playground.

Let's do a jigsaw puzzle

Let the child select the puzzle that suits him.

"Notebook" of Fabrics

Here is a simple and satisfying activity for a child with limited abilities. Gather a small stack of fabric with interesting colors, designs and textures, and then punch a hole in each piece of fabric. Secure the stack with a ring.

Materials: Fabric pieces or wallpaper; glue or a frayed-ends product such as Fray Check™ from Dritz; ring or clip; optional: reinforced holes.

Instructions:

1. Collect interesting fabric or wallpaper from resale shops, upholstery shops and fabric shops.
2. Have the child choose fabrics that appeal to her.
3. Cut swatches of the same size. Use pinking shears to cut fabric or fix the edges by brushing them with a 50-50 glue and water solution or with a frayed-ends product.
4. Use a hole-punch to make a hole in a corner of each swatch. Optionally, put a reinforced hole over the swatch holes.
5. Put the swatches on a ring.

Visual Activity 3
Stained Glass Windows

Use rich colors of tissue paper on a contrasting background to simulate stained glass. Use a paper backing or, for a stunning effect, have the child tape the patterned tissue paper directly to his bedroom window.

Materials: Tissue paper and foil giftwrap in different colors; construction paper or card stock for the backing; tape or glue.

Instructions:

1. Select complementary colors of tissue paper and construction paper.
2. Double a piece of tissue paper and trim it to the desired size.
3. Fold the tissue paper several times and cut small notches along each folded edge.
4. Optionally, fold the paper in a different pattern and make additional notches. For example, to achieve a snowflake design, fold the paper in quarters, and then in half to make a triangle. Cut notches along the long edge of the triangle.
5. Open the tissue paper and spread it flat on the construction paper. Tape or glue it in place.
6. Optionally, add more layers of notched tissue paper in different colors so that the patterns overlap. Make the notches in the top layers larger than the bottom so that the layers show through.

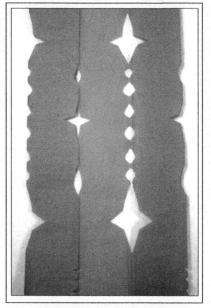

To make patterns for stained glass, fold paper multiple times and cut notches along the folds.

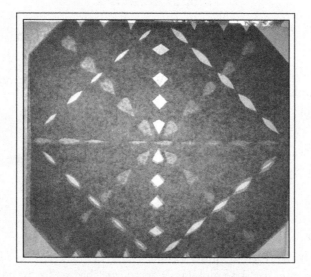

This stained glass window effect is tissue paper cut in patterns and taped to a window. Two layers of each color are used to intensify the colors. The two colors of tissue paper were cut into different patterns.

Visual Activity 4
Hand Weaving

Hand weaving is an example of a sensory immersion activity that can be the seed for a full-blown hobby. This weaving can be done in paper or fabric. The example shows an eight-inch (20 cm) weaving on a 12-inch (30 cm) background; you can make it any size.

Materials: Two complementary pieces of cloth, ribbon or paper; scissors or pinking shears (for fabric); school glue; cardstock or heavy paper for a backing; optional: clipboard.

Instructions:

1. Have the child select two types of paper, fabric or ribbons that are appealing to her and look nice together. Consider using fabric with texture.
2. Backing:
   a. Cut a 12-inch square of heavy paper or cardstock for the backing. This will be used to secure the weaving while it is worked on.
3. The vertical strands (the warp) are cut & within ½-inch of the bottom edge.
   a. Cut an eight-inch square of paper or cloth for the vertical strands.
   b. Cut the paper in vertical ribbons ½-inch (1.5 cm) wide, stopping ½-inch (1.5 cm) before the edge, as shown.
4. Horizontal ribbons (the weft):
   a. Cut strips of paper or cloth ½ x 8 inches (1.5 x 20 cm) wide.
5. Glue or tape the bottom edge of the warp to the bottom edge of the backing. Optionally, clip the background onto a firm board, table or notebook to make weaving easier.
6. Weave the strips or ribbons into the warp.
7. Adjust the strips so they are even. If using ribbons, you can let them hang off each side like fringe.
8. Dab bits of glue between the surfaces to hold the strips or ribbons in place at the edges.

Paper weaving using several different colors of paper.

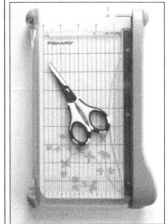

An inexpensive paper cutter makes the job easier, but scissors lets the child practice fine motor skills.

Visual Activity 5

Paper Strip Butterfly

Cutting paper strips and gluing them in pleasing arrangements stimulates the "line detectors" in the child's visual cortex and will make this activity a favorite.

Materials: Colored sheets of paper, magazines, scrapbook paper, wrapping paper or fabric, thin ribbon, or yarn; scissors; glue; paper, line drawing of an interesting shape (butterfly shape is in the Appendix.)

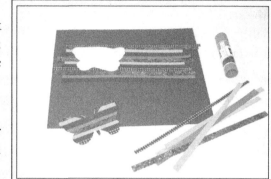

Instructions:

1. Cut narrow ribbons of paper or fabric as well as other materials such as cord or yarn. Make them longer than your chosen image.
2. Glue the ribbons side-by-side on a piece of paper. Let them dry.
3. Turn the paper over and draw the shape, making sure the ribbons run through the entire cut-out.
4. Cut out the shape.

Mosaics for Line and Detail

Mosaics stimulate the sense of vision with color and detail. You can use any simple shape as the subject of a mosaic. In this section, three different techniques are employed, graded for small children through teens. See *Touch activity 5* for another example.

Visual Activity 6

Layered Shapes

This activity can be done by a very young child if he is assisted with the cutting. Three pears are cut out using different colors of paper. The three pears are cut and layered on top of each other. The first pear, the bottom layer, remains uncut. The second pear, the middle layer, has a small piece cut out of its left side. The third layer, the top piece, has a larger section cut from it, most of the left side and part of the center.

To get the perspective correct, make the left section the brightest and lightest color, and the right side the darkest color.

Materials: The pear shape (in the Appendix), or another simple shape that you choose; colored paper, giftwrap, and scrapbook paper; scissors, glue; optional: cardstock, glitter or glitter glue.

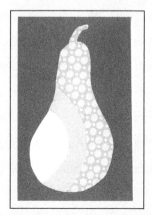

Instructions:

1. Cut out three copies of the pear in three different colors. Leave the shape with the lightest color whole. You will remove sections from the other two pears.
2. The pear has four lines for cutting. Choose the lines that match the photo. If you are using another shape, mark the lines for removing sections on the top two shapes (as described above).
3. Cut out the pieces to be removed from the top layers of the pear.
4. Glue the layers together.
5. Optionally, glue the finished work to a "frame" (a piece of construction paper).

138

Visual Activity 7
Large-Piece Mosaic

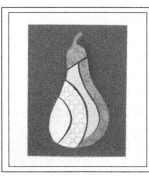

Cut the pear (or a shape of your choosing) into differently colored pieces, and put them back together like a jigsaw puzzle with or without the background showing through.

Materials: Same as for Activity 6. The pear shape is in the Appendix.

Instructions:

1. Cut out a copy of the pear and then cut it into five pieces using the lines drawn on the pear shape.
2. Using the five pieces for patterns, re-cut the pieces in five different colors.
3. Small children can glue the pieces back together on a piece of paper.
4. Have older child trim the pieces a little smaller to make a mosaic look, as in the photo.
5. Glue the pieces to a sheet of paper, leaving thin spaces between them for the background to show through.
6. Optionally, glue the mosaic to a paper frame.

In this version of the pear, we trim the pear pieces to leave space for the background to show. Cardstock was used for the "frame".

Visual Activity 8
Small-Piece Mosaic

Here is the same pear that was used in the previous two activities. This time the sections are filled in with small—sometimes very small—pieces of cut paper tiles.

The instructions for this project can be found in chapter 11, Multiple-day projects.

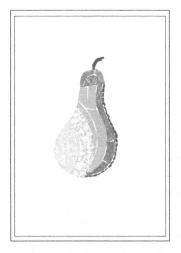

This mosaic uses very small tile pieces in the two leftmost sections of the pear. The remaining sections have larger tiles. The right border and stem is made of tiny black tiles.

Notebook Cover

Here is a fun visual immersion activity for creative children and teens: a cover for a binder or a folder.

Materials: Contrasting fabrics; several colors of construction paper; cardstock or cardboard; optional: picture of dog in the Appendix, or pictures from the internet or magazines; glue; scissors.

Instructions:

1. Select a piece of stiff paper, cardstock or cardboard for a backing. Cut it to fit the notebook. Set it aside.
2. Have the child design the cover using pictures or patterns she draws or finds on the internet or in magazines. Optionally, have her create a design using her name, or an image such as the dog in the Appendix (see photo).
3. Cut out the shapes and letters in colors and patterns that appeal to the child.
4. Glue the pieces onto the backing and attach them to the notebook.

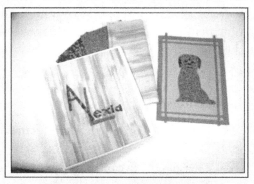

Two covers. Left: The cover background is a tie-dye fabric. The name Alexia has been cut out of contrasting fabric and glued to it. Right: The dog image was cut out of fabric and decorated with contrasting pieces of felt. The dog and a construction paper frame were glued to the front of the child's folder.

Mobiles for Movement

Some children crave visual movement. Have them create a simple mobile, and then see if they are ready for more complex ones. Start by using small objects such as the paper squares (see activity 10) or small object such as game tokens from an old Monopoly™ set. An older child can do all of the work. A younger child will need help assembling the mobile.

Visual Activity 10
Simple Mobile

This easy mobile has hanging letters of the child's name. But use any small objects in place of the letters.

Materials: Paper; string or cord; thin dowel rods; snippers, scissors; a hook for hanging the mobile; glue.

Instructions:

Create the objects to hang from the mobile

1. Cut out pieces of colored or patterned paper 2 x 4 inches (5 x 10 cm).
2. Fold the paper rectangles in half, making squares. Glue the sides together and let dry.
3. Punch a hole in a corner of each square.
4. Decorate the squares with letters, cutout pictures or designs.

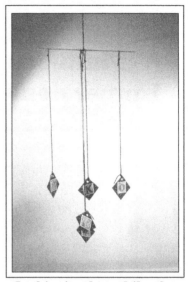

In this simple mobile, the hanging objects are paper squares with the letters of the child's name.

Create the mobile (See the photo)

1. Cut two dowel rods 12 inches (30 cm) or longer.
2. Cut the cord for hanging the mobile to the hook. The cord's length is the distance from the hook to where you want the dowel rods, plus a few extra inches (eight cm, or so) for attaching the two dowels together. (See below and the photo.)
3. Make a loop on one end of the cord. This will be used to hang the mobile on the hook.
4. Lay the two dowel rods crosswise on a table and wrap the cord crisscross three times at their intersection. Tie the cord tight. Optionally, place a drop of glue on the knot. Snip the short loose-end of the cord.

Make cords for the hanging objects

1. Cut cords in different-sized lengths. The cords in the photo vary from 18-23 inches (48-60 cm). This includes three inches (eight cm) for a loop and a knot at the ends.
2. Tie a loop at the end of each cord large enough to easily slip onto a dowel rod.
3. Thread the other end of the cord through a square and make a knot of the two strands.

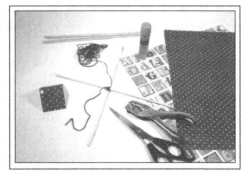

Wrap cord crisscross around the dowel rods three or four times. Knot cord tightly.

Hang the mobile

1. Attach the hook for the mobile in place (from a ceiling, doorway, bunkbed, etc.). Hang the dowel onto the hook from the cord's loop.
2. Hang the pieces. To arrange the mobile pieces on the "branches" of the mobile so they balance, use this technique: Hang a paper square onto whichever branch tilts highest. Repeat this step until all paper squares are in place. To level a tilted branch, do this: If a branch is tilted upward, move the squares closer to the end. If it is tilted downward, move it closer to the center.
3. Place a drop of glue on each cord where it sits on the dowel. Do this quickly, so that if the weight of the glue changes the balance of the mobile, you can adjust the squares before the glue dries.

Visual Activity 11

Multi-Sensory Immersion Project: Fruit Scented Mobile

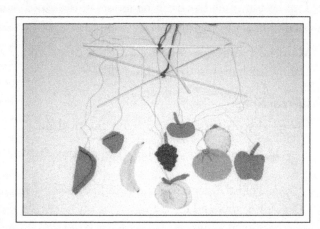

Once you have the "hang" of making a mobile, consider this multi-layered, scented fruit mobile. It is a project that can be done over a period of several days or weeks. The instructions can be found in chapter 11. Designs for the pieces of fruit are in the Appendix.

The instructions for this project can be found in chapter 11, Multiple-day projects.

Visual Activity 12

Carrel for Visual Distraction

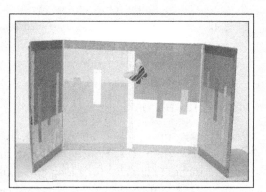

Here is a fun, practical project, a soft colored study-carrel to put on a desk at home or in school. The carrel is made of calming soft blues and greens and decorated with a single butterfly. This project will take the child several hours to complete, and so it is a practical visual immersion task for a child. About carrels: Carrels provide a visually quiet space for the child to work. This is helpful to children who are easily distracted.

The instructions for this project can be found in chapter 11, Multiple-day projects.

Visual Activity 13

Collage

The collage project is the ultimate visual immersion exercise. The child can select the colors and shapes, as well as the materials. For the child who likes things "just so," follow the instructions below. Otherwise, let the child use her creativity to make this picture her own. Does she want to pick real flowers, dry them for a week between the pages of a fat dictionary and then add them to the picture? Lovely idea! Does he want lions' heads for flowers? Great idea! How about rockets in the sky? Perfect! Find pictures of lions or rockets in a magazine and cut them out or hand draw the images onto the background.

The instructions for this project can be found in chapter 11, Multiple-day projects.

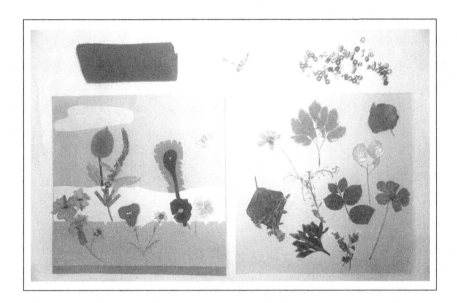

Other activities

For the precocious or creative child, consider these additional types of visual immersion activities:

1. Abstract doodling: 10-15 minutes of spirals, feathers, mazes
2. Make a mask
3. Scrapbooking
4. Photography of interesting images.

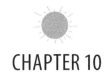

CHAPTER 10

Intense Movement

Immersion in Movement

Rigorous exercise has repeatedly been shown to increase attention-to-task and to reduce unwanted behaviors in the classroom in typical children and in children with ADHD. In addition, exercise has been shown to decrease anxiety. In this chapter, we present immersion in movement which involves a form of rigorous exercise called high intensity interval training (HIIT).

HIIT is a short, intense exercise program typically performed a few times a week. Examples of HIIT include the popular seven-minute workout programs. This chapter features FUNtervals, a four-minute, story-based version of HIIT. Children use fun exercises to act out the events in stories such as looking for buried treasure or going to the zoo. They alternately exercise for 20 seconds and rest for 10 seconds over a period of four minutes.

Four FUNtervals are presented in this chapter. Each is easy to perform and most important can be done in a small space such as a classroom. They are a viable way for teachers (or anyone) to help regulate children who are off-task or hyperactive. Following the four FUNtervals stories is an activity to "build your own" FUNterval.

FUNtervals were developed and studied for effectiveness by Canadian kinesiologist, Jasmine Ma. The name FUNtervals is appropriate; they are truly fun. Studies show that when they are performed regularly, children are more productive in the classroom and show decreased unwanted behaviors. FUNtervals can be done at home and in other settings, as well.

FUNtervals instructions

Each FUNterval features eight exercise periods, each followed by a rest period. If a story contains four exercises, children will repeat them twice for a total of eight. Eight-exercise routines are done once. The FUNterval called *Rock Paper Scissors* has a single exercise routine that is performed eight times. Its instructions are given separately. Here are general instructions:

1. Read the story's introduction to the children.

2. If the story is new to them, describe and practice the exercises.

3. Read the first section of the story.

4. Act out the story with the exercise:
   a. Perform the exercise for 20 seconds.
   b. Rest for 10 seconds and read the next section of the story.

5. Repeat step four until the story is complete.

6. If the story has four steps, repeat the entire routine.

Be sure to keep up a steady pace: 20 seconds of exercising and 10 seconds of resting without any other breaks. Children should go fast enough to achieve an aerobic workout, but not so fast that they lose control of their movement and their ability to self-regulate.

Safety Considerations: All exercises are done in place, but make sure that children have enough room to jump and land safely. Children with poor coordination should be positioned near a wall and with extra room to prevent bumping into others or falling.

Easy Workout FUNterval: Popcorn

The story: It's time for popcorn! It's movie night at the school and you have been asked to make the popcorn. You need to get it, pop it, scoop it into bags and quickly run it down to the cafeteria as fast as you can. Ready?

Instructions: Do each of the four exercises for 20 seconds, and then rest for 10 seconds. Try to do 20 reps of each step. That's one repetition per second. **Do the popcorn set twice.**

Considerations: This is appropriate for children of all ages. Shorten the length of time and the number of repetitions for very young children.

The exercises:

1. **Story:** "Reach to get a bag of popcorn from the top shelf and squat to put it into a cart. Can you get 20 bags?"

    Instructions:
    With your feet flat on the ground, reach high to get popcorn, and then squat with your arms out in front to put it onto the cart. Go fast!

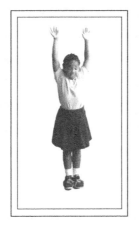 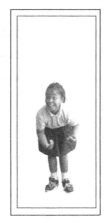

2. **Rest!** 10 seconds.

    Story: "Next, you need to pop the popcorn. Jump into the air with the popcorn kernels!"

    Instructions:
    Do jumping stars: jump in the air with arms and legs open

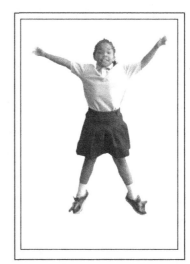

3. Rest! 10 seconds.

Story: "The popcorn is ready. Scoop up an armload and throw the popcorn into a sack."

Instructions:
Squat with your arms out front, and then jump up and toss arms to one side. Switch sides with each toss. (Alternately, toss in front rather than side-to-side.)

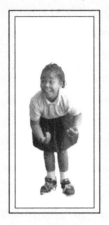 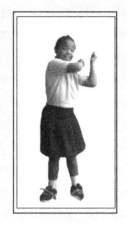 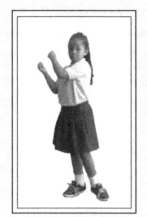

4. Rest! 10 seconds.

Story: "Run with the sack to the cafeteria!"

Instructions:
Run in place with knees high and arms swinging.

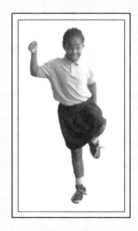 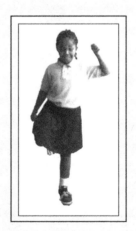

5. Rest! 10 seconds.

Story: "Your popcorn was a huge hit, everyone wants more! Repeat the steps! Can you make more than 20 bags?"

Instructions:
Repeat the steps one more time.

Easy Workout FUNterval: Zoo Animals

The story: Look out! Animals from the zoo have found a hole in the fence and escaped. Your job is to lead them back home once the fence has been mended.

Instructions: Follow the steps below and do each exercise for 20 seconds at a quick pace. Then rest for 10 seconds. When you have completed all eight steps, stop.

Considerations: This is appropriate for children of all ages. Shorten the length of time for very young children. Have children with poor balance stand near a wall for the monkey and koala moves. Make sure there is extra room for poorly coordinated children to jump.

The exercises:

1. Hop with the kangaroos back to their woodland!
    – Hop fast with arms bent at the elbow and your hands in fists.

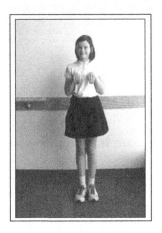 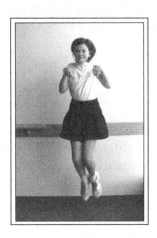

2. Rest! 10 seconds.
Grab branches and swing through the trees to lead the monkeys back home.
    – Lean to one side and raise the arm on that side to grab a branch. Stretch with the opposite leg. Now switch sides and continue to swing from one side to the other. (Have children stand near a wall or hold onto a chair, if necessary. Do this slowly with young children or children with poor coordination until they are able to assume the pose smoothly and switch from side-to-side.)

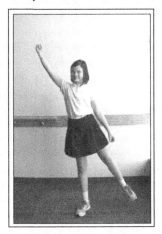 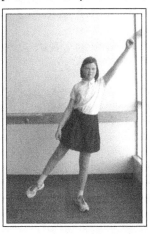

3. Rest! 10 seconds.

The koalas are up in the trees. Climb the trees to bring them down.

– Climb by raising one arm and the opposite leg at the same time. Now switch sides. (Do this slowly with young children or children with poor coordination until they are able to smoothly assume the pose and to switch from side-to-side.)

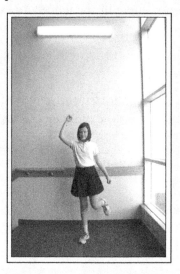 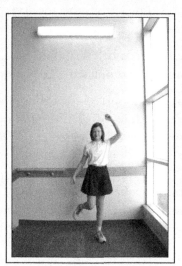

4. Rest! 10 seconds.

You need to lead the giraffes back home, but they are busy looking at children playing. Jump high to get the giraffes' attention.

– Power jump: bend over, and then jump as high as you can with arms and legs apart.

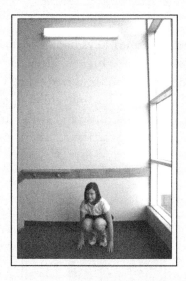 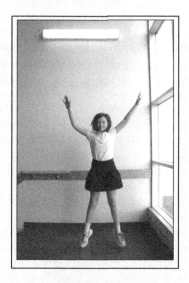

5. Rest! 10 seconds.

The bear cubs are sitting in a garden watching the bees—hoping to find a hive with honey. Squat down and pick up each bear. How many bear cubs can you pick up? Go fast before the bees swarm!

   – Squat down and scoop up with the arms. Try to pick up 10 or more cubs.

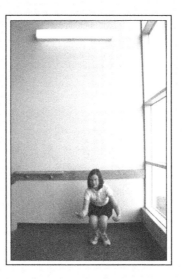

6. Rest! 10 seconds.

The penguins are making a beeline to the community pool. Waddle fast to lead them back to their ice house!

   – Waddle by keeping arms straight, lifting one leg and leaning to the opposite side. Quickly switch to the opposite side. Waddle fast!

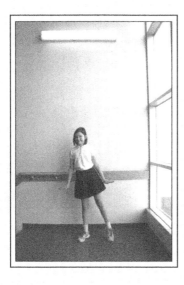 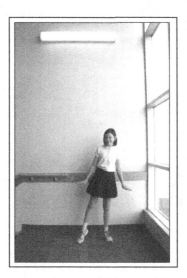

7. Rest! 10 seconds.

   Bring the frogs back to their lily pads. How fast can you hop?

   – Squat down with legs apart. Put hands on the floor with arms between the legs. Now hop in place. Keep hopping!

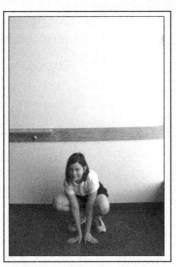

8. Rest! 10 seconds.

   Can you outrun the lions as you lead them back to their grassland? Don't get caught!

   – Run in place with knees high and arms swinging.

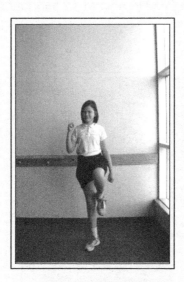 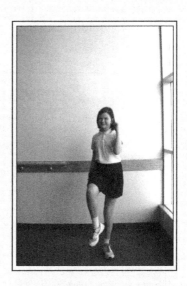

All done.

Medium Workout: Rock Paper Sissors Dance

The instructions for *rock, paper, scissors* are different than instruction for the other FUNtervals. It is a single exercise routine with three parts: crouch (rock), jump into a star (paper), and stand straight and reach (closed scissors). This routine is repeated for the entire 20 seconds. During the rest period, the child performs the hand movements for the *rock, paper, scissors* game. The rock, paper, scissors exercise is repeated for each of the eight exercise periods.

The story: There is a new beat and a new dance! It's called the rock paper scissors dance. Boom, boom, bop! Boom, boom, bop! Crouch, star, jump! Crouch, star, jump! How fast can you do the rock paper scissors dance? Can you do 10 crouch, star, jump-and-claps in a row?

Instructions: Repeat the three steps—rock, paper and scissors—in one constant motion and at a quick pace for 20 seconds. Then rest for 10 seconds. Do the dance eight times.

Considerations: This is appropriate for most children. Take care with small children. Try it first in a safe location where the child can land safely if she falls.

The exercises:

1. Crouch down small like a rock.
  – Squat on the ground with your elbows resting on your knees and your fists in a ball.

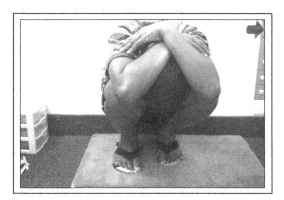

2. Jump up into a flat paper star.
  – Jump in the air with arms and legs open.

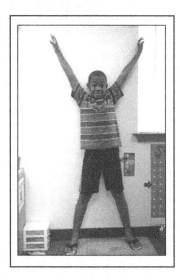

3. Close the scissors by bringing hands and feet together with a jump.

– Jump up while bringing your hands and feet together.

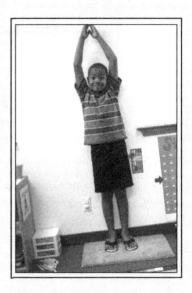

4. Relax and rest! 10 seconds.

– Play the traditional rock paper scissors game with a partner while you rest. Keep track of how many wins you get.

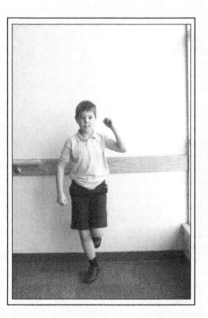 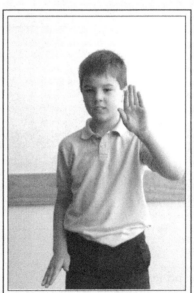 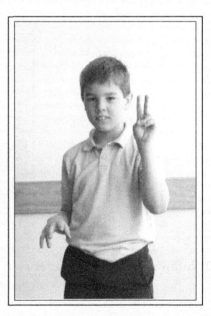

Do the dance eight times.

Stretch Workout: Pirate Treasure Hunt

The story: You found a map of an island with a big "X" on it. Is treasure buried there? Find out! Sail to the island, follow the map and dig for treasure!

Instructions: You will need a chair for this exercise. Follow the steps below and do each exercise for 20 seconds as fast as you can. Then rest for 10 seconds. When you have completed all eight steps, stop.

Considerations: Older children should be able to do these exercises. There are three types of challenges in the Pirate Treasure Hunt. Many of the eight steps have two-part movements and so the child will need to follow a sequence of two-four steps. The second is that although the movements aren't physically difficult, they cross midline, which can be challenging for younger children and children with special needs. The third challenge is that many exercises switch from side to side, and so the child has to quickly manage reverse movements. This last challenge is easily handled by having children not switch, but stay on the same side for 10 seconds, and then switch to the other side for the remaining 10 seconds.

The exercises:

1. Paddle your boat out of port onto the high seas! A pirate has seen your map. Go fast!
  – Sitting in a chair, twist the body from side-to-side as you quickly move arms in a paddling motion. You will be raising the arms over the shoulder, and then across the body and down (into the water), and then straight up to do the opposite motion.

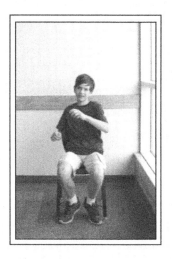 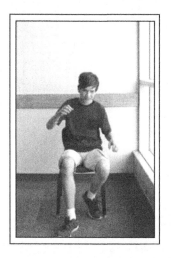

2. Rest! 10 seconds.
  You are in the high seas and the waves are huge! Lunge from side to side to keep balance. Jump when someone shouts, 'Big wave'!
  A. Lunge: Stand with legs far apart. Lean to the right and move your arms to that side. Put your right hand on your right thigh to help stabilize. Shift sides to reverse all the moves. Keep a steady pace, but do not go fast.
  B. The leader calls out, "Big wave!" every so often. Do a power jump by bending over, and then jumping as high as you can with arms and legs apart.

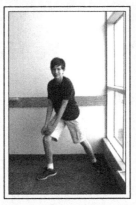 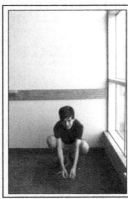 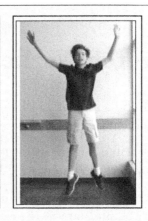

3. Rest! 10 seconds.

Man the sails! It's time to adjust the sails. Reach up to grab a sail and then stretch it to the opposite side to tie it down, and then grab another sail on the opposite side and tie it down.

- Place feet apart. Reach up high to the right side, and then stretch into a lunge to the left side by stepping out with the left leg. As you do this, move the arms down and over to rest on the left knee (for stability). Do this in a single smooth movement. Switch sides and repeat. Keep a steady pace.
- To make this easier, do the exercise on one side for 10 seconds, and then switch to the other side for the remaining 10 seconds.

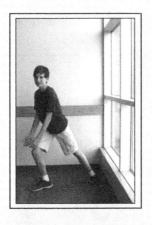 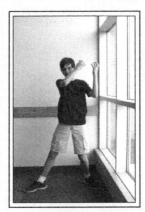

4. Rest! 10 seconds.

You see pirates in the waters behind you! Fire your cannons and duck for cover.

- Stand and put arms out in front, as if to light a fuse. Crouch down with hands over your ears, and then jump up and relight the fuse.

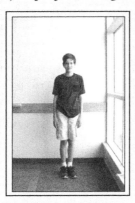 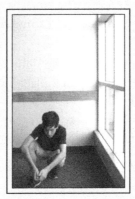 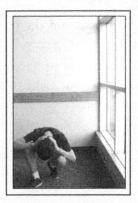

5. Rest! 10 seconds.

The pirates fire back! Crouch on the ground, then power jump to dodge their cannonballs!

    – Dodge, and then power jump.

    A. Dodge: Squat on the ground with your hands over your head.

    B. Power jump: Rise up, swing arms back and jump as high as you can with arms and legs apart.

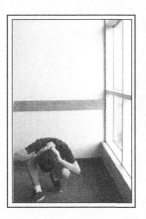 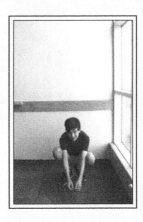 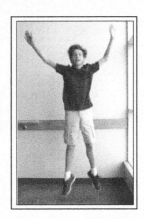

6. Rest! 10 seconds.

You have finally reached the island. Run off the ship and follow the map to the treasure spot.

    – Run in place with knees high and arms swinging.

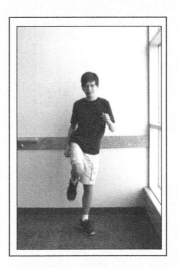

7. Rest! 10 seconds.

You have followed the map and now you see stones on the ground in the shape of an X. Dig deep. Is the treasure still there?

    – Bend and dig to one side, and then toss arms (with dirt) over the opposite shoulder. Switch from side to side as you dig. Alternately: Do this for 10 seconds, and then switch sides and dig on the other side for another 10 seconds.

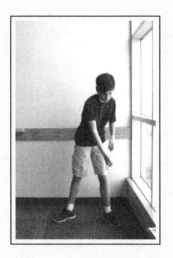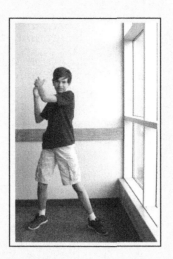

8. Rest! 10 seconds.

Hooray! You find a treasure chest. Inside is one gold doubloon for each jump you make.

– Jumping stars: Jump in the air with arms and legs open. 20 seconds.

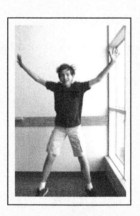

All done.

Make Your Own FUNterval

All types of stories and events can be cast into a FUNterval routine. You can choreograph movement to favorite cartoons (Dora and Boots, Teenage Mutant Ninja Turtles); fairy tales (*Rapunzel, The Three Little Pigs*); fables and nursery rhymes (*The Hare and the Tortoise, Old King Cole*); and sports scenarios (football, swimming or basketball).

If you are working with small children, select simple exercises. Older children can (and will enjoy) more challenging exercises.

Keep the story short. Pick just a few elements of interest to act out with exercises. You will need four or eight exercises for your story. Have the children help to create the choreography.

Begin the story with a warmup such as running in place or flying. Include a mixture of body movement such as stretching arms (reach or push); bending knees (lunge or squat); fast movement (running in place, jumping, or jumping stars); and crossing midline (digging, tossing, paddling, and so on).

Here are photo examples of movements to include in your story:

Fast movement: Jump, run, jumping stars

You can also include marching and climbing.

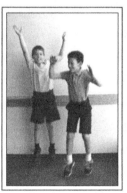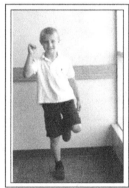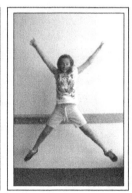

Stretch Arms: Scissors, fly, reach

Have children do each exercise on both sides of the body. For the scissors movement, the child will step or jump from side to side. For flying, she will alternately fly to the right and then to the left. Simple movements like reach can be implemented in two step routines, such as reach and relax.

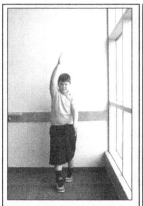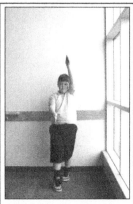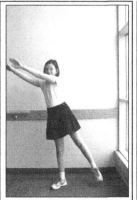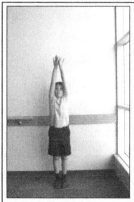

Knees: side lunge, and squats with arm movement

Below are examples of side lunges and squats. You can also include lunges with and without arm movement and side lunges with arm movement. An example of a lunge is shown in the gym exercises further below.

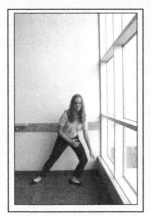 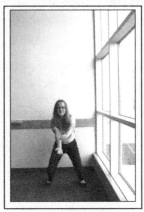

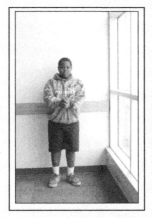 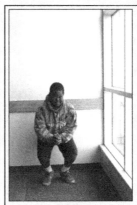 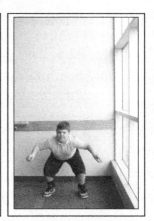

Cross midline exercises: paddling, pulling a lawn mower

Also include activities such as chopping wood and digging, as well as exercises such as windmills.

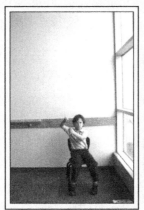 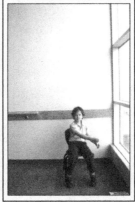 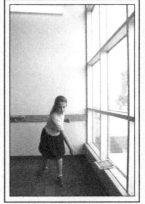 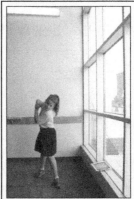

In a gym, you can add other types of exercises

In a gym setting, you can also include traditional exercises to your story.

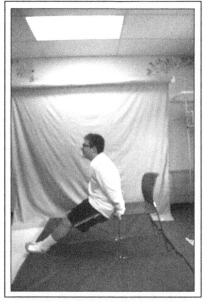

Triceps dip. Start in the position shown, with arms and legs fully extended, and then bend your elbows and knees. This will cause your body to dip below the level of the chair seat.

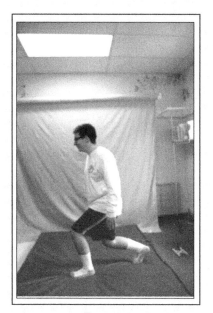

Lunge.

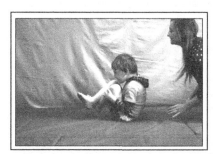

Cracked egg. Change between two positions, the cracked egg (shown), followed by relaxed arms and legs.

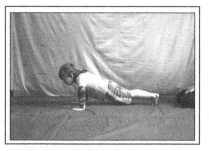

Pushups. Do either knee pushups or full pushups. Have the child go slow and rest when he's tired.

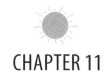

CHAPTER 11

Multi-Day and Multi-Sensory Projects

This chapter has the instructions for projects that can span a few days to a few weeks. Some of the projects are also multi-sensory.

Small-Piece Mosaic

Create a mosaic pear by gluing small—sometimes very small—pieces of cut paper tiles onto the entire surface.

This activity requires a great deal of patience. Consider doing it over a period of several weeks as an intervention for attention-to-task, attention-to-detail, and patience as well as for visual immersion.

Materials: A drawing of a shape (the pear shape is in the Appendix); colored paper, giftwrap, and scrapbook paper; scissors, glue; Optional: cardstock, glitter or glitter glue.

Instructions:

1. Make a copy of the pear (or a shape of your choosing).
2. Cut squares (or irregular pieces) of five colors of paper. To get the perspective correct, make the left section the brightest and lightest color, and the right side the darkest color. See the photo caption for ideas.
3. Glue the tiles on the drawing, occasionally mixing colors to make it fun and interesting.
4. Optionally, glue the mosaic to a paper frame.

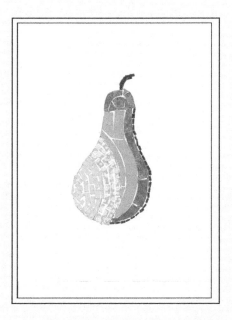

**This mosaic uses very small tile pieces in the two leftmost sections of the pear.
The remaining sections have larger tiles. The right border and stem is made of tiny black tiles.**

Multi-Sensory Immersion Project: Fruit-Scented Mobile

This activity creates a two-tiered mobile with scented fruit-shaped objects hanging from the branches. This is a multi-day project in which "fruit" can be made over a series of days. You can increase the sensory immersion by adding scented essential oil to the fruit while the work is in process.

The mobile has two unconnected tiers with four "branches" each. Each tier is independent and hangs from the same hook with one tier hanging lower than the other. If you wish to use just one tier, make longer rods to accommodate the fruit or use less fruit.

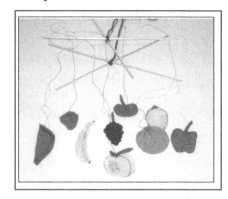

There are nine fruit shapes to choose from. You will want to use at least one piece of fruit for each "branch" of the mobile. If you use two tiers, as in the photo, you will need a minimum of eight pieces of fruit. Multiple pieces of fruit can be hung on a branch, and fruit can also be hung at the center where the two dowel rods meet. The fruit is attached to the branch with thread.

If you are adventurous and patient, you can alter the design and hang tiers from the branches of other tiers. This will be quite exciting to look at and provide a wonderful sensory break for a child who seeks visual movement.

Materials: *The fruit:* Colored felt or wool; scraps of cotton, silk, linen or wool; fruit shapes (in the Appendix); needle and thread; several different fruit-scented essential oils. *The mobile:* String or cord; thin dowel rods; snippers, scissors; a hook for hanging; glue.

Instructions:

Making the scented fruit

1. Make a copy of the fruit shapes you plan to use. Cut them out.
2. For each piece of fruit: Trace the shape onto felt or wool and cut out two copies (for front and back).
3. Cut scraps of green felt for the stems, rind and leaves on the fruit. You will need front and back trim for rinds and small button ends of the watermelon, strawberry, orange and lemon. You only need one stem for the grapes, apple, cherry and peach. Glue the trim in place.
4. If you are using a wool felt or wool fabric for the fruit, put the two copies of each shape together and glue them lightly (neatly) at the edges.
5. Otherwise, first place a scrap of natural fabric (cotton, linen, wool or silk to hold the scent) between the two copies of the shape, and then glue them neatly at the edges.
6. When the fruit has dried, make thread hangers:
   a. Cut thread in doubled lengths varying from 30-40 inches (76-100 cm), or at a pleasing finished length plus three inches (10 cm) for a loop and a knot at the ends.
   b. For each piece of fruit, use a needle to draw a thread through the top of the piece of fruit. Tie the ends in a knot.

Make the mobile

If you are making two tiers, make each separately. Remember to make the cords for the lower tier longer than those for the upper tier. When you hang the second tier, adjust the fruit so they are pleasant to look at.

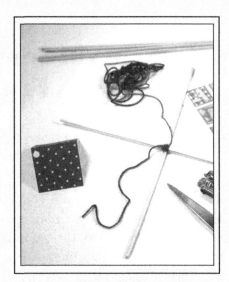

Create the mobile (See the photo)

1. Cut two dowel rods 12 inches (30 cm) or longer.
2. Cut the cord for hanging the mobile to the hook. The cord's length is the distance from the hook to where you want the dowel rods, plus a few extra inches (eight cm, or so) for attaching the two dowels together. Add an additional few inches if you plan to make two tiers. (See below and the photo.)
3. Make a loop on one end of the cord. This will be used to hang the mobile on the hook.
4. Lay the two dowel rods crosswise on a table and wrap the cord crisscross three times at their intersection. Tie the cord tight. Optionally, place a drop of glue on the knot.
5. If you are making two tiers, leave a few inches (8 cm, or so) of cord between the tiers. Then repeat step 4 to add the second tier. Snip the short loose-end of the cord.

Wrap cord crisscross around the dowel rods three or four times. Knot cord tightly.

Hang the mobile

1. Attach the hook for the mobile in place (from a ceiling, doorway, bunkbed, etc.).
2. Hang the dowel onto the hook from the cord's loop.
3. To arrange the mobile pieces on the dowel rods so they balance, use this technique: Hang a piece of fruit onto whichever branch is tilted highest. Repeat this process until all pieces of fruit are in place. To level a tilted dowel, do this: On a section that is tilted upward, move the fruit closer to the end. If it is tilted downward, move it closer to the center.
4. Place a drop of glue on each thread where it sits on the dowel. Do this quickly, so that if adding the glue changes the balance, you can adjust the pieces of fruit slightly.
5. Once the glue has dried, repeat this process for the second tier.

Add the scent

1. Each day or so, place a drop of essential oil at the center of each piece of fruit.

Multi-Day Project 3
Carrel for Visual Distraction

Create a soft colored study-carrel to put on a desk at home or in school. The carrel is made of calming soft blues and greens and decorated with a single butterfly. This project will take the child several hours to complete, so it serves as visual immersion for a child who also needs calming.

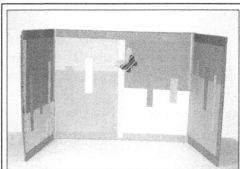

Materials:

- A 3-fold science project board;
- A variety of paper such as construction paper, gift wrap and scrap booking paper in different shades of soft blues and greens. Use paper that is solid in color or has soft, abstract prints. It is important that there is nothing in the decoration that will distract the child;
- School glue or several glue sticks;
- Scissors and, optionally, a paper cutter;
- Butterfly shape (in the Appendix);
- Packing tape, colored duct tape or decorative tape to bind the carrel edges and folds.

You will also need a large enough work area and a place to store the paper and partially completed carrel between steps.

Instructions:

Let the glue dry between steps so that previous work does not become spoiled.

1. Shorten the 3-fold board to the appropriate height using a utility knife.
2. If the backside of the 3-fold board is unattractive, cover it with colored paper. Do not cover the folds (they need to move).
3. Lay the 3-fold board flat and lay out the different styles of solids and prints on it until you find a pleasant arrangement.
4. Cut the background pieces to fit the entire surface of each of the three panels. Glue them in place. Do not paper over the top of the folds.
5. Use decorative tape to bind the edges on all four sides. Optionally, cover the edges with strips of paper and bind them with clear packing tape.
6. Lay the carrel flat and put decorative tape along the folds.
7. Cut strips for the decoration using varied papers and glue them in place.
8. To make the butterfly, use the shape in the Appendix. Cut it out and glue it in place.

Collage With or Without Dried Flowers

The child can select the colors and shapes, as well as the materials. For the child who likes things "just so" follow the instructions below. Otherwise, let the child use her creativity to make this picture her own. Does she want to pick real flowers, dry them for a week between the pages of a fat dictionary and then add them to the picture? Lovely idea! Does he want lions' heads for flowers? Great idea! How about rockets in the sky? Perfect! Find pictures of lions or rockets in a magazine and cut them out or hand draw the images onto the background.

Remember to keep a cup of water and a towel nearby for those who do not like gooey materials.

Materials: Cardstock for the backing; green and blue paper or paint for the sky, grass and hill; scraps of colored paper and fabric for the clouds, flowers and other objects, glue and scissors; optional: dried flowers and small leaves; cut out colors or pictures from magazines; decoration such as beads and glitter glue.

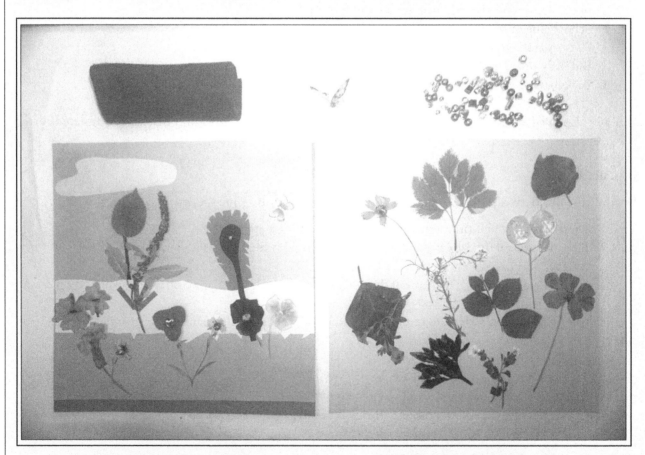

Left: Materials include bright felt, a paper butterfly and beads.

Right: Flower and leaves were carefully flattened and dried.

Drying the flowers:

1. Collect small flowers and leaves.
2. Place them in a large heavy book such as an encyclopedia. Put the book in a safe place where it will not be disturbed. If possible, add additional heavy books on top to increase the weight. Let the flowers and leaves dry in the book for a week or two.
3. Delicately remove them from the book and place them on flat surface where they will not be disturbed.

Construction:

1. Create the grass, hill, and sky from layers of construction paper. Lightly glue them together.
2. Add clouds, sun and tree trunks.
3. Make other objects for the collage such as drawn flowers, along with fun things such as lions' heads, giant frogs or rockets.
4. Add cut-out images from magazines.
5. Arrange the objects on the collage and glue them in place.
6. Add beads, glitter and other decorations.

Multi-Sensory Immersion Project: Dish Garden

Here is a project with many different sensory components: desensitization to touch and immersion in touch as the child coats a dish in sand and pebbles; visual immersion through sorting colored pebbles and making a pattern with them; and the sensory aspects of the plants themselves. You can select plants with scents, for example, the spaghetti sauce group of basil, oregano, parsley, rosemary and parsley or a prickly touch grouping of cactus plants, soft-to-the touch plants like moss or fuzzy purple passion plant, or frilly plants that give the eyes soft stimulation such as a spider fern or the coleus.

Making the Pot

Materials: Medium-large glass dish 3" or more deep; sand; glue; contrasting colors of pebbles, popcorn, beans or tiles; small tub larger than the bowl; cardstock or index cards for the stencil; optional: varnish and brush. Plants such as moss (touch), mint (smell), coleus (visual).

Instructions: First, glue a light covering of sand onto the bowl, dry it and then glue on the pebbles. If you plan to put a name or pattern on the bowl, put those pebbles first and put the background pebbles on last. When the bowl is completely covered and dry, optionally cover it with 50-50 mixture of glue and water or have an adult varnish it.

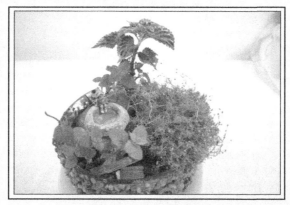

Planter contains mint (scent) moss (touch) and coleus (visual).
They were planted in potting soil and have a woodchip covering. Pebbles would work, too.

You will be working sections of the bowl (whatever lies flat at the top) one at a time. If the bowl is round you may be limited to putting pebbles on just 2-3 inches at a time. Beyond that, the bowl angles too much causing the glue to run and the pebbles to fall.

The bowl sits in sand in a tub so that the section to be worked on is level.

Instructions:

Stabilize the bowl: To keep the bowl steady and level as you work with it, put sand in the tub, turn the bowl on its side and lightly bury the bottom in sand.

Glue sand on the bowl: To help the pebbles to adhere, glue sand on the bowl as a first layer. Work on the section of the bowl that is on top and is reasonably flat. Turn the bowl and continue gluing sand on it. Let the section you worked on dry for several hours and then continue until complete.

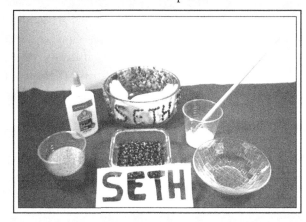

Create a pattern: If you plan to put a pattern or name on the bowl, create a stencil for your pattern. As an example, if you are putting a name on the bowl, draw it in block letters on the cardstock, and then carefully cut out the insides of the letters.

Put the pattern or name on the bowl: Carefully position the stencil on the bowl and put glue in a small portion of the stencil. Lift the stencil and carefully place pebbles on the glue. Work only on level sections of the bowl so that the glue and pebbles do not run. Let that section dry before proceeding.

Cover the background in pebbles: Once the pattern is dry, you can begin to glue in the background pebbles. Again, make sure that the glue does not run and pebbles do not slide.

(Optional) Varnish the bowl: To waterproof the bowl for use as a planter, have an adult cover the pebbles with one or more layers of varnish or another waterproof covering.

Planting the dish garden

Material: pebbles; potting soil; small fragrant plants such as basil, rosemary, dill (or seeds and peat pots to grow them).

The process using small plants: Place ½ inch of small pebbles in the dish for drainage. Fill the bowl to within 1 inch of the top with potting soil. Place small one or more small plants in the soil and firmly tamp them down. Make sure to leave 3-4 inches between plants to allow them to grow. Water the plant and place it in a sunny window or under a grow light.

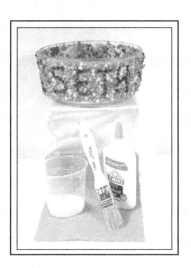

Monkey Yarn Doll with Cap

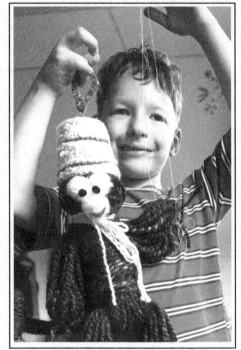

Here is a multi-day project constructed of easy steps for the child with construction assistance from an adult. The monkey is made of yarn balls and wrapping. His hat is made of yarn chains glued to a plastic cup. His head, body and hat are held together with wire (either a hanger or picture-hanging wire) which extends into a tail. The doll's face is decorated with buttons, pipe cleaner and felt. Decoration is optional. The inventive therapist, teacher or parent will think of alternate methods for constructing and decorating the yarn doll, as needs dictate. The finished monkey, including hook, is approximately 20 inches (50 cm) tall. The measurements given are actual, but feel free to modify them for a different appearance.

The finished monkey.

Monkey materials: One skein of yarn, plus other colors of yarn for face and for ties; wire or pliable wire hanger, tape for ends of wire; corrugated cardboard or other firm material cut in strips for wrapping; 4 or more 12-inch (30 cm) pipe cleaners in a complementary color; decorations like ribbons, beads, felt for eyes, nose and mouth; glue.

Hat materials: A small-medium size paper or plastic cup (author used 3 inches (7.5 cm) diameter at the brim, 3 inches (7.5 cm) tall); two skeins of thick yarn – different colors, plus scrap yarn of a third color (for the hat trim and ties); white school glue; bowl of water to wash glue off finger tips.

Step 1: The hat

The child will be wrapping and gluing yarn chains or thick yarn around the surface of the cup and also making a spiral on the cup bottom. Optionally, the child can first make chains of the yarn and then glue it.

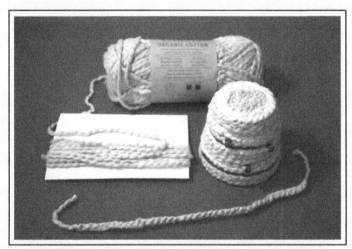

1. (Adult) Pierce a hole in the bottom center of the cup for the wire to pass through (during the construction phase).
2. Make a yarn chain long enough to wrap around the cup once or twice.
3. Pull each end of the chain tight and snip off the yarn ends close to the chains.
4. Glue the chain around, starting at the top rim.
5. Make additional chains in the three different colors and glue them onto the cup in a striped pattern. Tuck the ends in and glue them.

Create the hat by gluing yarn to the side and the bottom of a plastic cup. The yarn can be simply wrapped on the cup or it can be chained first.

6. To cover the bottom of the cup, make a short chain and roll it into a spiral. Glue it at the center of the cup bottom. Add one or two rows of chain of another color on the outside edge of the cup bottom and glue it.

7. Let the hat thoroughly dry before handling.

Step 2: The monkey's head

Roll yarn into a ball for the head. It should be sized so that the cup can sit on the head as a cap – (approximately 10 inches (25 cm) in circumference.) Cut the yarn, leaving an extra 10 inches on the end. It may be needed for adjusting the size of the head. Dab bits of glue under the top layer of yarn to keep it from unrolling.

Step 3: Connect hat and head (adult)

1. Gently push the wire through the ball of yarn so that it extends for 13 inches (34 cm).

2. Push the hat onto the wire.

3. Bend the wire and thread it through the cap again, leaving a two inch (5 cm) loop at the top of the hat. Pull apart the hat and head so that you can twist the two wires together inside the hat at the top, making the hat secure.

4. Bend the wire loop on top of the hat into a circle.

5. Push the raw end of a pipe cleaner into the hole in the cup and wrap it tightly three times around the base of the wire loop.

6. (Child) Wrap pipe cleaner around the loop wire. Use additional pipe cleaners, as needed. Trim and bury the raw ends of pipe cleaner.

7. Push the head up the wire to the hat, gently pushing the raw wire end into the head as you do so, so that it is safely inside the center of the head.

8. Pull the head and hat tight together and then softly bend the wire so that they (hat and head) remain tight while the rest of the monkey is constructed. (The wire will need to be re-straightened later.)

9. Set aside.

Step 4: Make arms and legs

1. Wrap yarn on a 13 inch (34 cm) strip of cardboard. (Wrapping bulky yarn 14 times produced arms that were four inches (25 cm) around.)

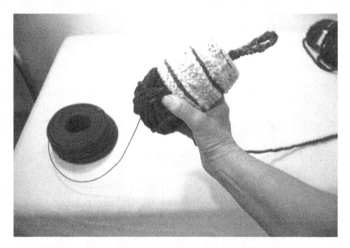

Wire is gently pushed through the yarn ball and through the top of the hat. It is then bent and looped back through and the raw end is hidden in the yarn ball. The loop sticking out of the hat is wrapped with a pipe cleaner.

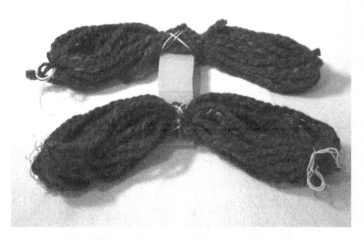

Lash the arms and legs onto the ends of the cardboard strips using scarp yarn.

2. Use small pieces of yarn for ties. Put a tie through each end of the wrapped yarn (through the loops of yarn) and tie it securely. Slip the arms off of the cardboard.

3. Repeat for the legs.

Step 5: Attach the arms and legs

1. Cut two strips of corrugated cardboard 6.5 x 2 inches (17cm x 5 cm). Place them back to back. (The wire will slip through these during the construction phase.)

2. Lay the arms and legs in place at each end of the cardboard (see photo) and lash them to the cardboard by wrapping crisscross-style with scrap yarn.

Step 6: Make the body

Wrap yarn around the cardboard lengthwise and widthwise until the cardboard is completely covered and the body is the desired thickness—about 8.5 inches (22 cm) around the belly.

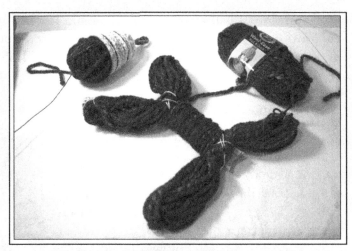

The head and body, ready for assembly.

Step 7: Connect the body, form the tail: (adult)

1. Read all Step 7 instructions before cutting the wire. Cut the wire to about twice the length of the body and tail. See photo.

2. Gently push the wire into the body between the two layers of cardboard.

3. Create the tail: Extend the wire about 13" (33 cm) out for the tail, then bend it, doubling back to the body. Trim it. (See photo.)

4. Slip about 2" (5 cm) back into the body (between the two cardboards). Twist the two tail wires together, leaving a small loop on the end for decoration.

5. Push the body snugly up to the head and then bend the tail to the side to keep it snug.

6. Wrap pipe cleaner tightly around the wires where the monkey's tail meets the body, burying the raw ends of pipe cleaner.

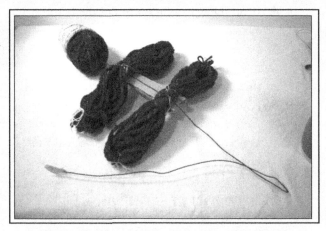

Wire is pushed between the two cardboard strips and is bent to form a tail. The end of the wire will be safely tucked back into the body between the cardboard strips.

Step 8: Make the tail

You will make a yarn tail the same size as the wire tail, attach it to the wire tail at both ends and then wrap both together (along the length) with more yarn. That is, you will wrap the yarn in circles around the whole length of the tail. Next, you will secure the body with pipe cleaner and decorate the end of the tail.

1. Wrap yarn seven times around the same card you used to make the arms and legs. Put ties around the yarn at each of the ends and remove the wrapped yarn from the card.

2. Use pipe cleaner to attach the yarn tail to the wire tail at each end of the tail. At the body end, wrap the pipe cleaner around the tail tightly, leaving extra pipe cleaner for later use.

3. Wrap yarn in small tight circles from one end of the tail to the other. Tie off the yarn and secure it to the tail.

4. Neatly wrap the ends of the tail with the remaining pipe cleaner. Bury the raw ends of the pipe cleaners.

5. (Optional) Decorate the end of the tail with additional tied-on scraps of yarn.

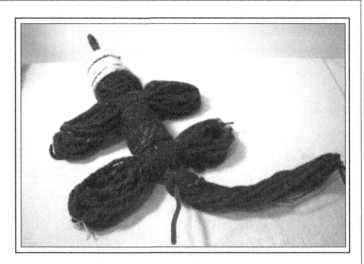

Yarn is wrapped onto the twisted wire tail and tied. Pipe cleaner is attached to the wire at both ends of the tail and wrapped several times over-top. Next the entire length of yarn and wire will be wrapped in yarn and secured with the remaining ends of pipe cleaner.

Face: There are many ways of finishing the monkey. Here are some possibilities.

1. Our solution: Roll three yarn balls for the eyes and mouth, occasionally adding a dab of glue to keep the yarn from slipping.

2. Glue three pom-poms or cotton balls together, as shown.

3. Simply add beads or button eyes and nose.

4. Glue on red yarn, bead or button for mouth, or twist on red pipe cleaner for mouth.

5. Anchor the face onto monkey's head using needle and thread. Optionally glue the face in place.

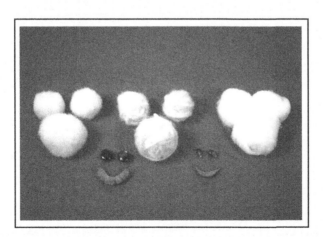

You can use pompoms, rolled-yarn balls or cotton balls for the face. Decorate them with beads or buttons for eyes and red felt or pipe cleaner for the mouth.

Bibliography

Abdollahian, E., Mokhber, N., Balaghi, A., & Moharrari, F. (2013). The effectiveness of cognitive-behavioural play therapy on the symptoms of attention-deficit/hyperactivity disorder in children aged 7-9 years. *Attention Deficit Hyperactivity Disorders*, 41-46.

American Academy of Pediatrics. (2011). ADHD: Clinical practice guideline for the diagnosis, evaluation, and treatment of attention-deficit/hyperactivity disorder in children and adolescents. *Pediatrics*, 1007-1022.

Bellefeuille, I. B., Schaaf, R., & Polo, E. R. (2013). Occupational therapy based on Ayres Sensory integration® in the treatment of retentive fecal incontinence in a 3-year-old boy. *The American Journal of Occupational Therapy* , 601-606.

Benson, T. M., Roley, S. S., Mailloux, Z., Parnham, L. D., Koomar, J., Schaaf, R., et al. (2014). Interrater reliability and discriminative validity of the structural elements of the Ayres Sensory Integration Fidelity Measure. *American Journal of Occupational Therapy*, 506-513.

Best, J. R. (2010). Effects of physical activity on children's executive function: contributions of experimental research on aerobic exercise. *Developmental Review*, 331-351.

Brown, N. B., & Dunn, W. (2010). Relationship between context and sensory processing in children with autism. *American Journal of Occupational Therapy*, 474-483.

Cerliani, L., Mennes, M., Thomas, R. M., di Martino, A., Thioux, M., & Keysers, C. (2015). Increased functional connectivity between subcortical and cortical resting-state networks in autism spectrum disorder. *JAMA Psychiatry*, 767-777.

Cerrillo-Urbino, A. J., Garcia-Hermosa, A., Pardo-Guijarro, M. J., Santos-Gomez, J. L., & Martinez-Vizcaino, V. (2015). The effects of physcial exercise in children with attention deficit hyperactivity disorder: a systematic review and meta-analysis of randomized control trials. *Child: Care, Health and Development*, DOI:10.1111/cch.12255.

Chang, Y., Owen, J. P., Desai, S. S., Hill, S. S., Arnett, A. B., Harris, J., et al. (2012). Autism and sensory processing disorders: shared white matter disruption in sensory pathways but divergent connectivity in social-emotional pathways. *PLOS One*, DOI: 10.1371/journal.pone.0103038.

Chen, T., Michels, L., Supekar, K., Kochalka, J., Ryali, S., & Menon, V. (2014). Role of the anterior insular cortex in integrative causal signaling during multisensory auditory-visual attention. *European Journal of Neuroscience*, 1-11.

Clauw, D., Arnold, L. M., & McCarberg, B. H. (2011). The science of fibromyalgia. *Mayo CLinic Proceedings*, 907-911.

Coates, J, Taylor, J. A., & Kayal, S. (2015). Parenting interventions for ADHD: A systematic literature review and meta-analysis. *Journal of Attention Disorders*, 831-843.

Donkers, F. C., Schipul, S. E., Baranek, G. T., Cleary, K. M., Willoughby, M. T., Evans, A. M., et al. (2015). Attenuated auditory event-related potentials and associations with atypical sensory response patterns in children with autism. *Journal of Autism and Developmental Disorders*, 506-523. Dunst, C. J., Meter, D., &

Hamby, D. W. (2011). Influences of sign and oral language interventions on the speech and oral language production of young children with disabilities. *CELL Reviews*, 1-20.

Fabio, R. A., Castriciano, C., & Rondanini, A. (2015). Auditory and visual stimuli in automatic and controlled processes. *Journal of Attention Disorders*, 731-740.

Faller, P., Hunt, J., van Hooydonk, E., Mailloux, Z., & Schaaf, R. (2015). Application of data driven decision making using Ayers Sensory Integration™ with a child with autism. *American Journal of Occupational Therapy*, doi:10.5014/ajot.2016.016881.

Garland, T. (2014). *Self-Regulation Interventions and Strategies*. Eau Claire, WI: PESI Media.

Grandin, T., & Panek, R. (2013). *The Autistic Brain: Thinking Across the Brain*. Boston: Houghton Mifflin Harcourt.

Greene, S. A., Hernandez, L., Tottenham, N., Krasileva, K., Bookheimer, S. Y., & Depretto, M. (2015). Neurobiology of sensory overresponsivity in youth with autism spectrum disorders. *JAMA Psychiatry*, 778-786.

Guderjahn, L., Gold, A., Stadler, G., & Gawrilow, C. (2013). Self-regulation strategies support children with ADHD to overcome symptom-related behavior in the classroom. *Attention Deficit Hyperactivity Disorders*, 397-407.

Hochhauser, M. E.-Y. (2010). Sensory processing abilities and their relation to participation in leisure activities among children with high-functioning autism spectrum disorder (HFASD). *Research in Autism Spectrum Disorders*, 746-754.

Hodgson, K., Hutchinson, A. D., & Denson, L. (2014). Nonpharmalogical treatments for ADHD: a meta-analytic review. *Current Perspectives*, 275-282.

Horst, J. S., Parsons, K. L., & Bryan, N. M. (2011). Influences of sign and oral language interventions on the speech and oral language production of young children with disabilities. *Frontiers in Psychology*, DOI: 10.3389/fpsyg.2011.00017.

Hoza, B., Smith, A. L., Shoulberg, E. K., Linnea, K. S., Dorsch, T. E., & Blazo, J. A. (2015). A randomized trial examining the effects of aerobic physical activity on Attention-Deficit/Hyperactivity Disorder symptoms in young children. *Journal of Abnormanl Child Psychology*, 655-667.

Ismael, N. T., Mische-Lawson, L. A., & Cox, J. A. (2015). The relationship between chilldren's sensory processing patterns and their leisure preferences and participation patterns. *Canadian Journal of Occupational Therapy*, 316-324.

Jordon, C. (2014, October 3). *Does the 7 Minute Workout Really Work?* Retrieved April 15, 2015, from The Johnson and Johnson Official 7 Minute Workout Blog: https://7minuteworkout.jnj.com

Kasparek, T., Theiner, P., & Filova, A. (2015). Neurobiology of ADHD from childhood to adulthood. *Journal of Attention Deficits*, 931-943.

Kinnealey, M., Pfeiffer, B., Miller, J., Roan, C., Shoener, R., & Ellner, M. L. (2012). Classroom modification on attention and engagement of students with autism or dyspraxia. *American Journal of Occupational Therapy*, 511-519.

Kirby, A. V., Little, L. M., Schultz, B., & Baranek, G. T. (2015). Observational characterization of sensory interests, repetitions and seeking behaviors. *American Journal of Occupational Therapy*.

Klika, B., & Jordan, C. (2013). High-intensity circuit training using body weight: maximum results with minimal investment. *American College of Sports Medicine Health & Fitness Journal*, 8-13.

Koenig, K. P., & Rudney, S. G. (2010). Performance challenges for children and adolescents with difficulty processing and integrating sensory information: A systematic review. *American Journal of Occupational Therapy*, 430-442.

Koegel, R. L., Bharoocha, A. A., Ribnick, C. B., Ribnick, R. C., Bucio, M. O., & Fredeen, R. M. (2012). Using individual reinforcers and hierarchical exposure to increase food flexibility in children with autism spectrum. *Journal of Autism and Developemental Disorders*, 1574-1581.

Koyuncu, A., Ertekin, E., Yuksel, C., Ertekin, B., Celebi, F., Binbay, Z., et al. (2015). Predominantly inattentive type of ADHD is associated with social anxiety disorder. *Journal of Attention Disorders*, 856-864.

Lane, A. E., Molloy, C. A., & Bishop, S. L. (2014). Classification of children with autism spectrum disorder by sensory subtype: a case for sensory-based phenotypes. *International Society for Autism Research*, 1-12.

Lees C, H. J. (2013). Effect of aerobic exercise on cognition, academic achievement, and psychosocial function in children: a systematic review of randomized control trials. *Preventing Chronic Disease*, DOI: 10.5888/pcd10.130010.

Longobardi, E., Spataro, P., & Rossi-Arnaud, C. (2012). The relationship between motor development, gestures and language production in the second year of life: a mediational analysis. *Infant Behavior and Development*, DOI: 10.1016/j.infbeh.2013.10.002.

Lucker, J. R., & Doman, A. (2015). Neural mechanisms involved in hypersensitive hearing: Helping children with ASD who are overly sensitive to sounds. *Autism Research and Treatment*, DOI:10.1155/2015/369035.

Ma, J. K., Le Mare, L., & Gurd, B. J. (2015). Four minutes of in-class high-intensity interval activity improves selective attention in 9- to 11-year olds. *Applied Physiology, Nutrition, and Metabolism*, 238-244.

Ma, J., Gurd, B., & Levesque, L. (2014, October 14). *Funtervals*. Retrieved April 15, 2015, from Queen's University: www.skhs.queensu.ca/musclephysio/Activity Booklet.pdf

Ma, J., Le Mare, L., & Gurd, B. J. (2014). Classroom-based high-intensity interval activity improves off-task behaviour in primary school students. *Applied Physiology, Nutrition, and Metabolism*, 1332-1337.

Makris, N., Liang, L. B., Valera, E. M., Brown, A. B., Petty, C., & Spencer, T. (2015). Toward defining the neural substrates of ADHD: A controlled structural MRI study in medication-naïve adults. *Journal of Attention Deficits*, 944-953.

May, T, Brewer, W. J., Rinehart, N. J., Enticott, P. G., Brereton, A. V., et al. (2010). Differential olfactory identification in children with autism and Asperger's disorder: A comparitive and longitudinal study. *Journal of Developmental Disorders*, 837-847.

May-Benson, T. A., & Koomar, J. A. (2010). Systematic review of the research evidence examining the effectiveness of interventions using a sensory integration approach for children. *American Journal of Occupational Therapy*, 403-414.

McGlone, F., Wessberg, J., & Olausson, H. (2014). Discrimination and affective touch: sensing and feeling. *Neuron Perspective*, 737-755.

McQuade, J. D., Vaughn, A. J., Hoza, B., Murray-Close, D., Molian, B. S., Arnold, L. E., et al. (2014). Perceived social acceptance and peer status differentially predict adjustment in youth with and without ADHD. *Journal of Attention Disorders*, 31-43.

Medford, N., & Chritchley, H. D. (2010). Conjoint activity of anterior insular and anterior cingulate cortex: awareness and response. *Brain Sturcture and Function*, 535-549.

Menon, V., & Uddin, L. Q. (2010). Saliency, switching, attention and control: a network model of insula function. *Brain Structure and Function*, 655-667.

Miller, L. J. (2011, November 16). Treatment of sensory modulation disorder. *SPD University*, www.spduniversity.org/2011/11/16/106.

Miller, L. J., Nielson, D. M., & Schoen, S. A. (2012). Attention deficit hyperactivity disorder and sensory modulation disorder: a comparison of behavior and physiology. *Research in Development*, 804-818.

Milte, C. M., Parletta, N., Buckley, J. D., Coates, A. M., Young, R. M., & Howe, P. R. (2015). Increased erythrocyte eicosapentaenoic acid and docosahexaenoic acid are associated with improved attention and behavior in children with ADHD in a randomized controlled three-way crossover trial. *Journal of Attention Deficits*, 954-964.

Miltenberger, C. A., & Charlop, M. H. (2014). Increasing the athletic group play of children with autism. *Journal of Autism and Developmental Disorders*, 41-54.

Parnham, L.D., Cohen, E.S., Spitzer, S., Koomar, J.A., Miller, L.J., Burke, J.P., & Brett-Greene, B. (2007). Fidelity in sensory integration intervention research. *American Journal of Occupational Therapy*, 216-227.

Pfeiffer, B. A., Koenig, K., Kinnealey, M., Sheppard, M., & Henderson, L. (2011). Effectiveness of sensory integration interventions in children with autism spectrum disorders: A pilot study. *American Journal of Occupational Therapy*, 76-85.

Reese, E., Sparks, A., & Leyva, D. (2010). A review of parent interventions for preschool children's language and emergent literacy. *Journal of Early Childhood Literacy*, 97-117.

Rosen, P. J., & Factor, P. I. (2015). Emotional impulsivity and emotional and behavioral difficulties among children with ADHD: an ecological momentary assessment study. *Journal of Attention Disorders*, 779-793.

Reynolds, S., Kuhaneck, H. M., & Bfeiffer, B. (2016). Systematic review of the effectiveness of frequency modulation devices in improving academic outcomes in children with auditory processing difficulties. *American Journal of Occupational Therapy*, DOI: 10.5014/ajot.2016.016832.

Schuck, S. E., Emmerson, N. A., AH, F., & Lakes, K. D. (2015). Canine-assisted therapy for children with ADHD: preliminary findings from the positive assertive cooperative kids study. *Journal of Attention Deficits*, 125-137.

Schaaf, R. C., & Mailloux, Z. (2015). *A clinician's guide for implementing Ayres Sensory Integration: Promoting participation for children with autism.* Bethesda, MD: AOTA Press.

Schaaf, R. C., Benevides, T., Mailloux, Z., Faller, P., Hunt, J., & van Hooydonk, E. (2014). An intervention for sensory difficulties in children with autism: A randomized trial. *Journal of Autism and Developmental Disorders*, pp. 1493-1506.

Schaaf, R. C., & Smith-Roley, S. (2006). *Sensory integration: Applying clinical reasoning to practice with diverse populations.* Austin, TX: Pro-Ed.

Small, D. M. (2010). Taste representation in the human insula. *Brain Structure and Function*, 551-561
Smith-Roley, S., Milloux, Z., Parnham, D., Schaaf, R. C., J, L. C., & Cermak, S. (2015). Sensory integration and praxis patterns in children. *American Journal of Occupational Therpay*, DOI: 10.5014/ajot.2015.012476.

Tamm, L., Nakonezny, P. A., & Hughes, C. A. (2014). An open trial of a metacognitive executive function training for young children with ADHD. *Journal of Attention Disorders*, 551-559.

Using individualized reinforcers and hierarchical exposure to increase food flexibility in children with autism spectrum. (2011). *Journal of Autism and Developemental Disorders.*

Wang, J. (2014, September 2). *The benefits of the 7 minute workout for kids.* Retrieved April 15, 2015, from North Shore Pediatric Therapy: nspt4kids.com/resources/exercise/The benefits of the 7 minute workout for kids/

Watling, R., & Hauer, S. (2015). Effectiveness of Ayres Sensory Integration® and sensory-based interventions for people with autism spectrum disorder: a systematic review. *American Journal of Occupational Therapy*, DOI: 10.5014/ajot.2015.018051.

Woo, C. C., & Leon, M. (2013). Environmental enrichment as an effective treatment for autism: A randomized controlled trial. *Behavioral Neuroscience*, 487-97.

Woo, C., Donnelly, J. H., Steinberg-Epstein, R. R., & Leon, M. (2015). Environmental enrichment as a therapy for autism: a clinical trial replication and extension. *Behavioral Neuroscience*, 412-422.

Woodward, T. W. (2009). A review of the effects of martial arts practice on health. *Wisconsin Medical Journal*, 40-44.

Yang, X., Carrey, N., Bernier, D., & MacMaster, F. P. (2015). Cortical thickness in young treatment-naive children With ADHD. *Journal of Attention Deficits*, 925-930.

Zwi, M., Jones, H., Thorgaard, C., York, A., & Dennis, J. A. (2011). Parent Training Interventions for Attention Deficit Hyperactivity Disorder. *Campbell Collaboration Library of Systematic Reviews, 8, 1-99. http://www.campbellcollaboration.org/lib/project/143/.*

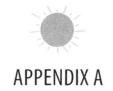

Books to Read with Children

This list is courtesy of Jean Walsh, MS, SLP. She recommends some great books to help young children develop sounds, vocabulary and humor.

Book	Author	Uses
The Baby Goes Beep	Parr, Todd	Baby, "b" words
There's a Bird on Your Head	Willems, Mo	"b" words
I Can Say That	Lederer, Suzy	Animal names and sounds, No, Hi, Bye
I Can Do That	Lederer, Suzy	Early verbs
I Can Play That	Lederer, Suzy	Early verbs
Have You Seen My Cat	Carle, Eric	Cat
That's Not My Puppy	Watts, Fiona	Puppy
Five Little Ducks	Raffi	Duck
Silly Sally	Wood, Audrey	Animals, humor
Napping House	Wood, Audrey	Animals, Repetition
Ten Little Fish	Wood, Audrey	Counting
Ten Apples Up On Top	Le Sieg, Dr. Seuss	Apples
My Car	Barton, Byron	Car
Who Stole the Cookies	Moffatt, Judith	Cookies
Bubble Trouble	Packard, Mary	Bubbles
Animal Kisses; Noisy Kisses; Peek-a-boo Kisses; Goodnight Kisses	Saltzberg, Barney	Kisses
Mrs. Wishy Washy	Cowley, Joy	Wash
Mrs. Wishy Washy's Christmas	Cowley, Joy	Wash, Cold
Smarty Pants	Cowley, Joy	Verbs
Meanies	Cowley, Joy	Early Verbs
Crunch Munch	London, Jack	Eat
Snuggle Wuggle	London, Jack	Hug
Splash	McDonnell, Flora	Hot
Where's Spot	Hill, Eric	Colors, animal sounds
Hand, Hand, Fingers, Thumb	Perkins, Al	Pair with a drum for Stop, Go using fingers and thumb
Bugs in Space	Carter, David	Bugs, humor
Give a Mouse a Cookie	Numeroff, Laura	Repetition, humor
Take a Mouse to School	Numeroff, Laura	Repetition, humor
Green Eggs and Ham	Dr. Seuss	Repetition, humor
Mix it Up	Tullet, Herve	Verbs, humor
Press Here	Tullet, Herve	Verbs, humor

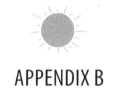

Illustrations

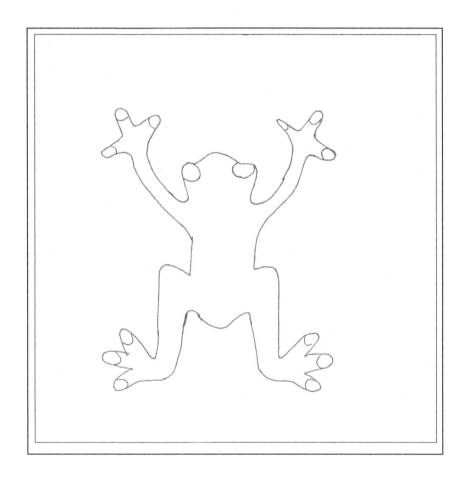

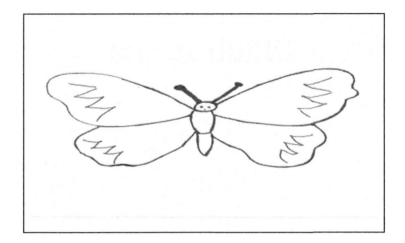

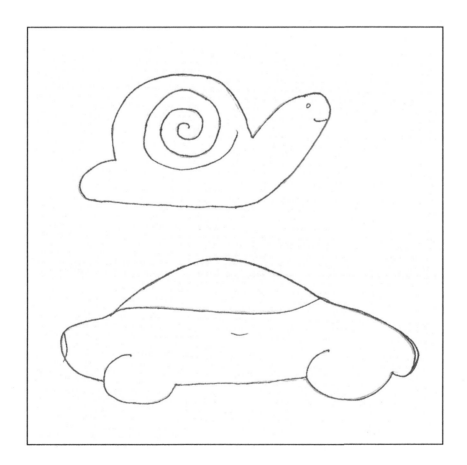

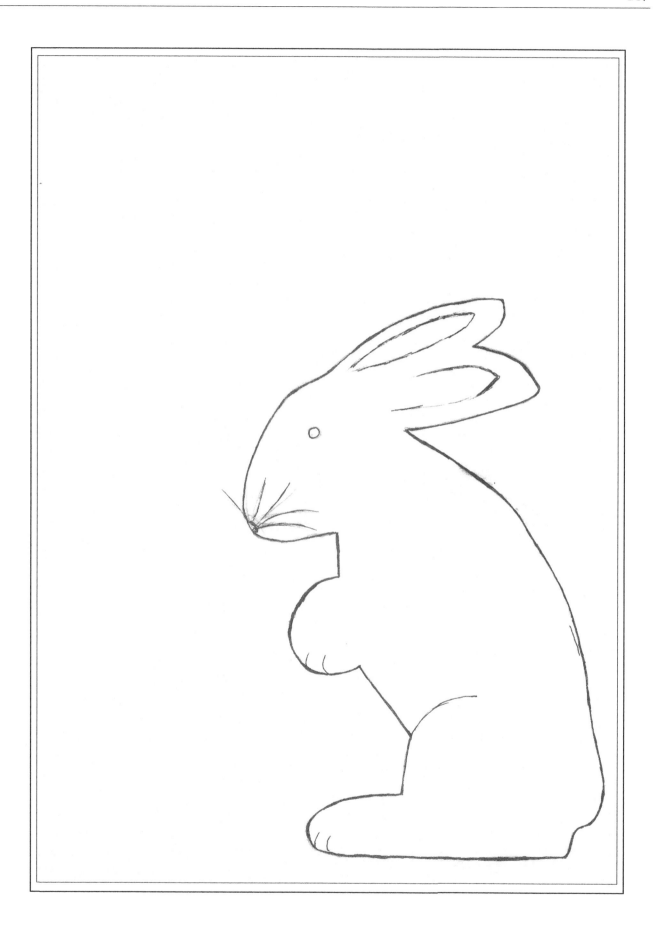

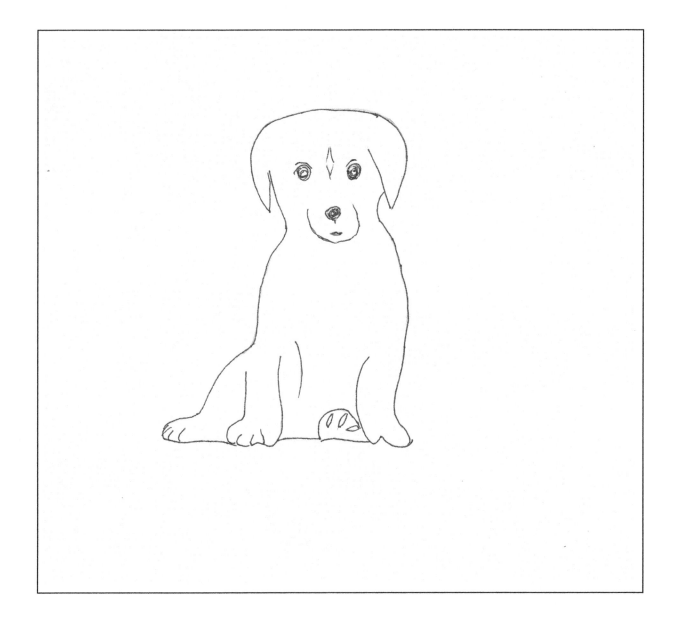

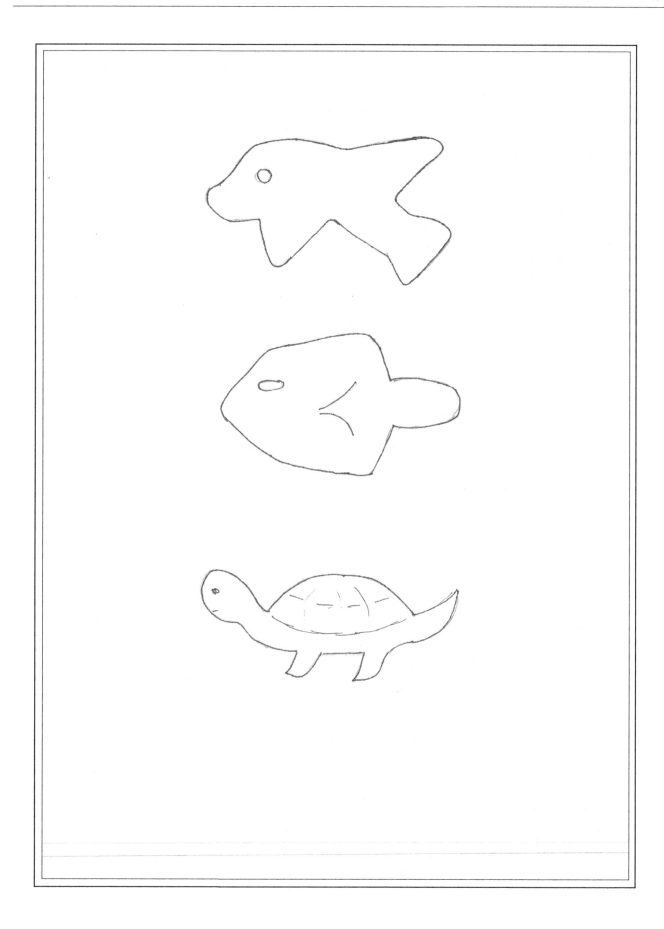

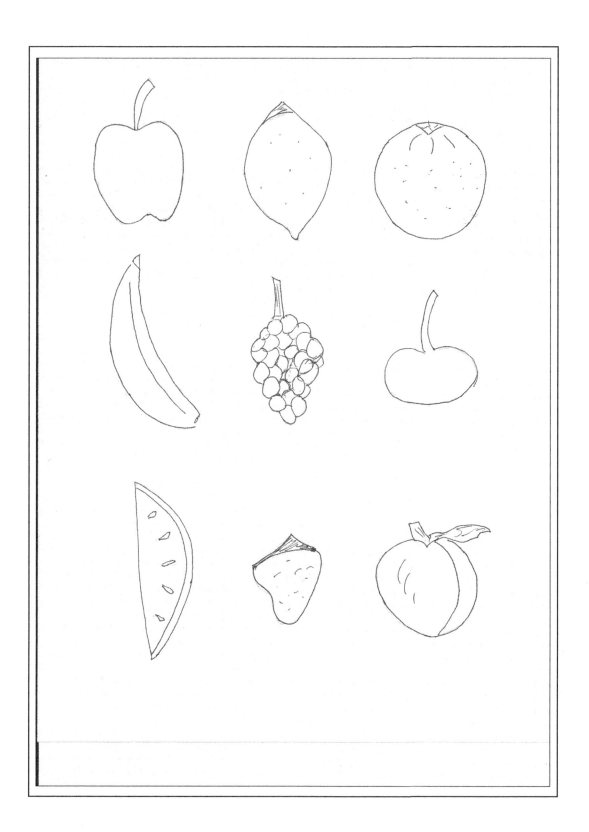

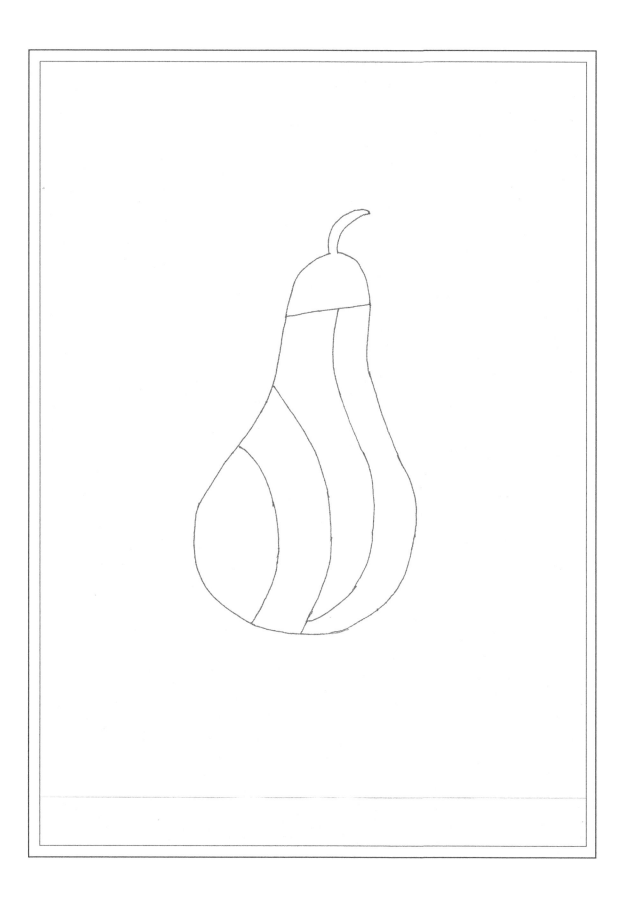

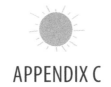

Activities by Name

Chapter 5: Enrichment Mix-Ins

Chapter 6: Touch

Chapter 7: Taste and Smell

Made in the USA
Las Vegas, NV
12 April 2022

47354565R00118